The Healing Benefits of Acupressure

Acupuncture Without Needles

The Healing Benefits of Acupressure

ACUPUNCTURE WITHOUT NEEDLES

F. M. Houston, D.C.

Keats Publishing, Inc. New Canaan, Connecticut

B260:1V Keats

THE HEALING BENEFITS OF ACUPRESSURE
Acupuncture Without Needles

Published in 1974 by Keats Publishing, Inc.
27 Pine Street (Box 876), New Canaan, Connecticut 06840

ISBN 0-87983-068-9
Library of Congress Catalog Card Number: 74-75986
Printed in the United States of America

To all the friends this book has made in the past
and to the new readers who seek the healing art

Contents

Foreword

by Linda Clark, M.A.

The world is in serious need of healing today and because of it, healing should not be reserved for a few select individuals, professions or specialists only. Everyone should have access to some self healing methods.

In the days of our forefathers, transportation was limited. Each family had its own natural remedies and methods of treating illness until the doctor arrived. As a result many a life was saved by such means and was approved by the doctor who often arrived to find the patient on the mend.

Today we have come full circle. Transportation is again limited. Few doctors make house calls. By all means, if you need one, find a qualified doctor if you can. If you can't, the alternative is to have ready, as did your ancestors, safe methods of treating or preventing illness. The Orientals, both doctors and peasants, have long used herbal and other safe home remedies handed down from generation to generation. One of these, *Acupuncture,* for doctors, or a similar do-it-yourself method known as *Shiatsu,* was and is used at home with great success. Now acupuncture is taking the whole world by storm. Yet few people can find a reliable acupuncturist.

Fortunately there is a do-it-yourself technique now made available to the public which you can learn in minutes and use on yourself or members of your family, safely. It is done, not by the use of needles, but with the fingertip applied to acupuncture points. Those who have tested it thoroughly report that it works. Doctors of all kinds (including M.D. s), registered nurses, physiotherapists and other professional therapists of many kinds are learning the technique, both for their own use as well as for their patients. This form of acupuncture, called *Acupressure,* may be slower and require more repetition, but it is free, simple to use and available night or day in your own home with very little effort on your part.

F. M. Houston, D.C., who has perfected this system for many years is teaching classes to eager professionals from coast to coast. Now for the first time he is making this exciting knowledge available to *you,* the public.

You do not have to attend classes unless you wish. You do not have to memorize anything. All you do is to look at the charts in this book, use your fingertip and press on the appropriate acupuncture point which relates to the disturbance which bothers you.

You cannot buy health once it is gone, but you can, if you know how, help yourself when it is slipping. To learn the technique, you have nothing to lose except the small cost of this unique book, which will become one of your most treasured possessions.

Introduction

In the late 1800's a famous French scientist named Michael Faraday, who invented the first electric motor, made a very profound statement, "All school children know that all matter is composed of atoms, vibrating at different rates of speed to form different densities; but what we should also know is that all matter or any substance—dense, liquid or gaseous—owes whatever power it may possess to the type of electrical charge or vibration given off by that substance."

Any good book on physics will tell you that energy cannot be destroyed but it can travel. It cannot be seen, since it is invisible, but it can leave the body and as it leaves we get weaker and weaker. The heart is the generator for the electricity in the body. If you have ever talked with anyone who has had a heart attack, he will tell you that his energy just seemed to drain away.

The body not only is electrical in nature, but it has its positive and negative poles. The heart represents the negative; the brain, right side, represents the positive. There should be balance between the heart and the brain.

Contact healing is a method of contacting the electrical centers in the body. Balance and order must be established before health becomes established. Acupuncture is a proven system used for centuries by the Orientals to create a smooth flow of vibratory energy throughout the body by contacting various points on the pathways which relate to various organs, glands and cells. The acupuncturist, of course, uses steel needles which are inserted at certain points identified with the various body areas and their disturbances. By changing their distorted vibrational nature, balance is restored and the body can repair itself.

Contact healing, or acupressure, also treats the various points of the body which relate to various areas, glands and organs. However, instead of using needles, this method is a do-it-yourself technique of pressing your fingertip on these contact points. If the organ, area or gland the point represents is in trouble, that point will be sore, indicating an energy leak at that exit.

Once you have located a painful spot, just put your fingertip on it, press firmly and hold it there. Do not move it, or you will move off of the zone which needs help. This pressure closes an energy leak. As soon as you close the leak, the polarity is reversed and the energy flows back into the part of the body which was losing it. You should feel a warmth build up in the organ you are treating and the warmth indicates that regeneration and repair are beginning to take place. When there is no longer any tenderness at the contact point you can feel assured that the regeneration is complete.

Acupuncture may, or may not, require more than one treatment. Contact therapy usually does need even more time. The reversal of symptoms in contact therapy seldom takes place in one treatment. But the more you treat and the longer you treat, the sooner the job is done to help you feel fit once again.

Please remember that this or any other method of healing does not cure anything! We can assist or work with nature, but nature herself is the real healer.

Since its inception in 1956, contact healing has spread to many countries, and many letters from this country and others testify to the fact that it is helpful therapy and that nearly anyone can use it with benefit.

I merely ask you to try it as others have done. I make no claims. You can be your own judge of the results. This is far more convincing than any promises I might make. I do say however, that if you wish to have success, you must be persistent. If your body has long been at odds with itself, the good results you are seeking may take more time than if your disturbance is recent.

At the very least the system is safe and simple and free. You have nothing to lose and much to gain if you will be consistent and faithful until you witness a restored feeling of well-being.

F. M. Houston, D.C.

The Pressure Points of the Body

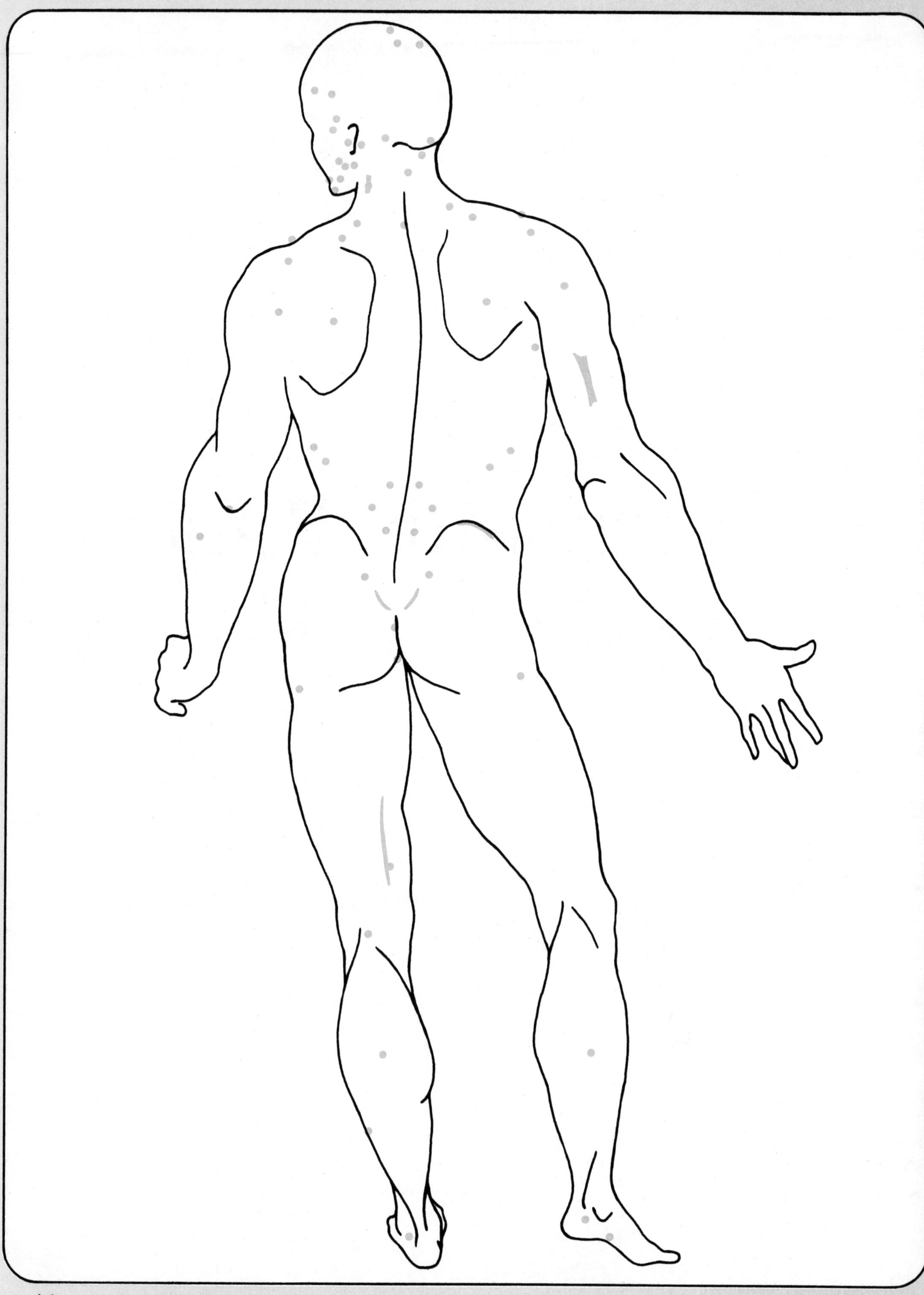

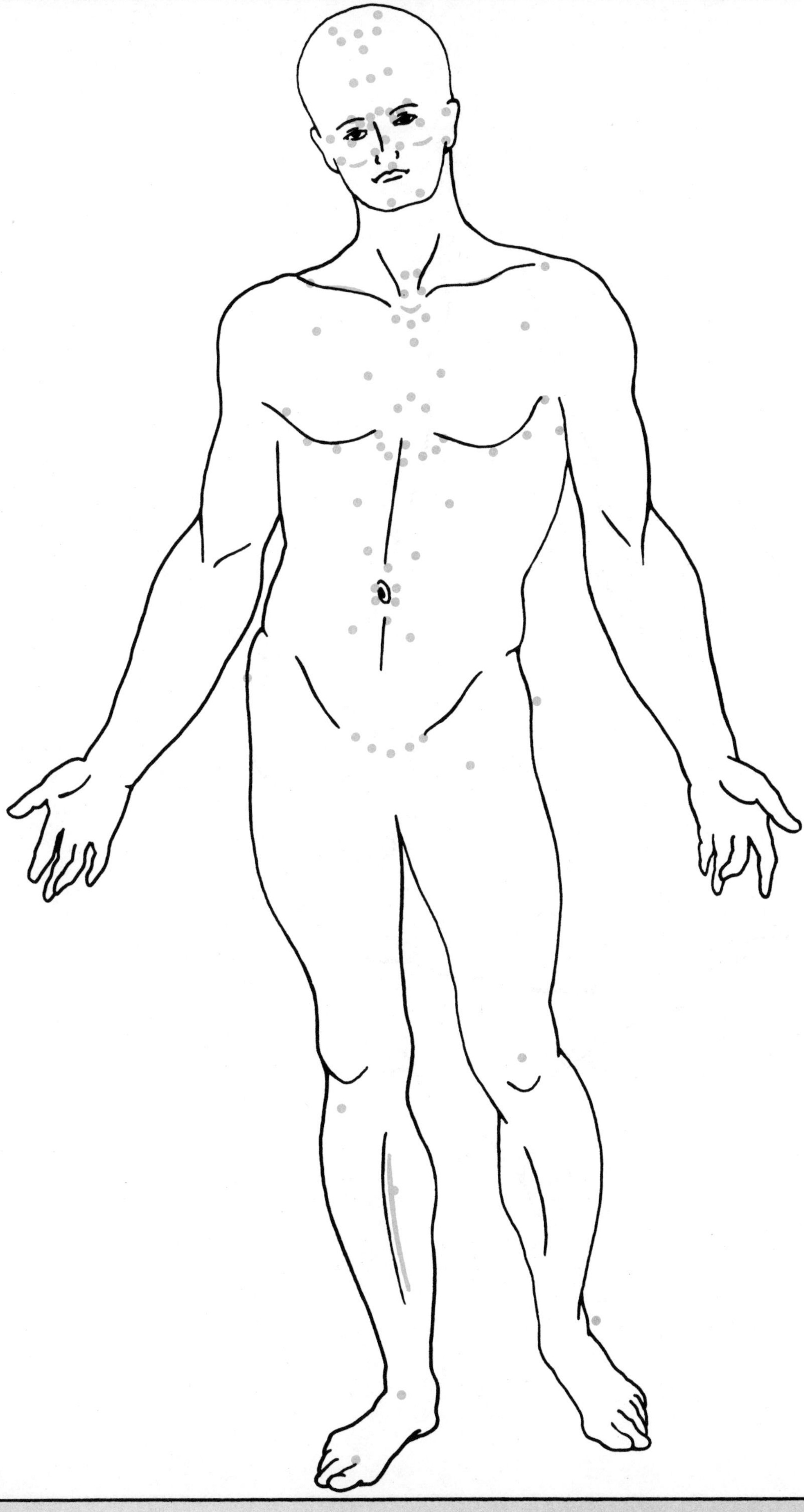

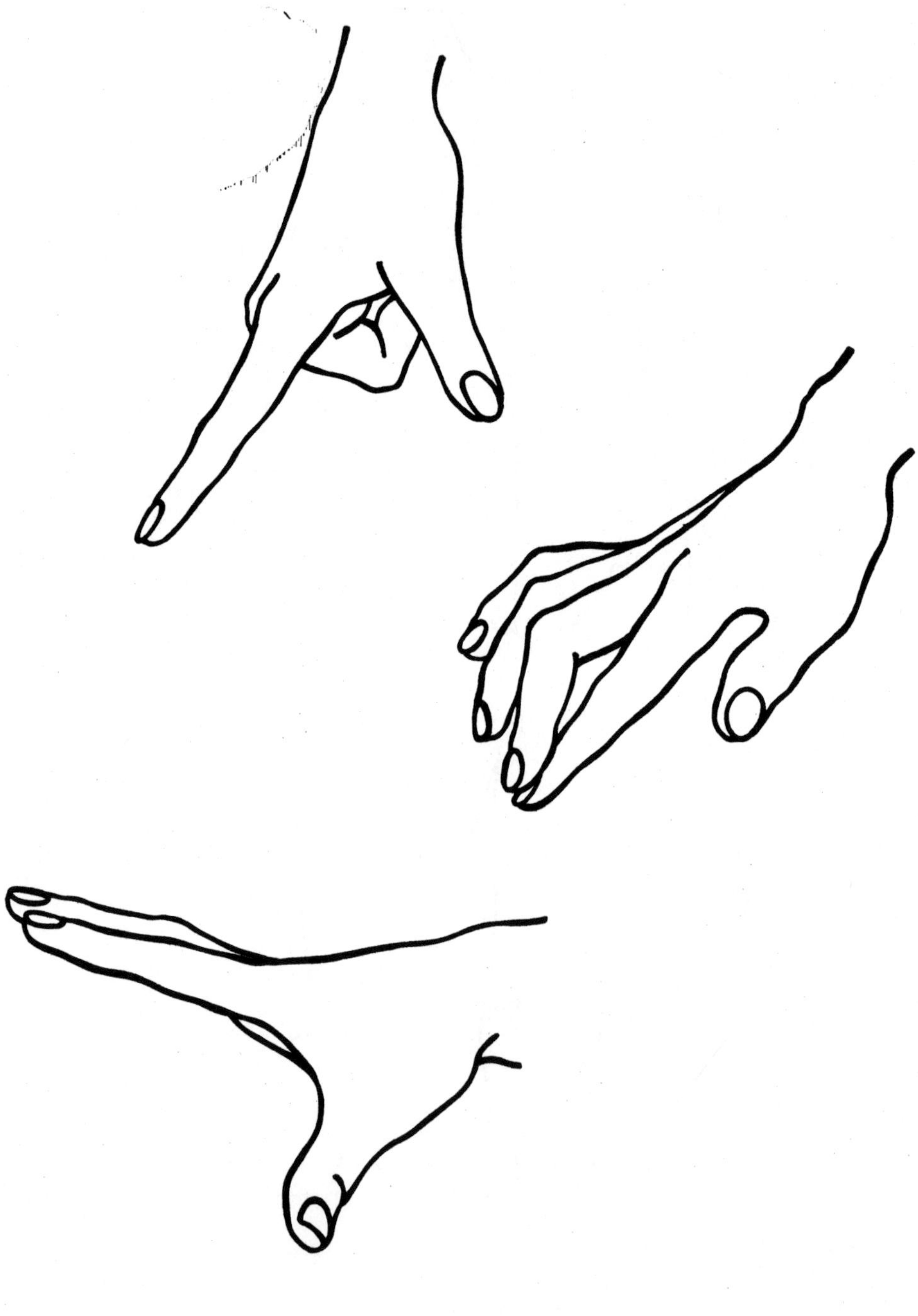

How To Treat the Pressure Points

How to Treat

By contacting any center on the head, face or body which is painful, you immediately begin helping that organ or tissue. For instance, if your knee hurts and there has been no accident or strain of any kind, and contact #43 (which treats the knee) is not painful, then the knee trouble may be a symptom only, perhaps of kidney trouble which you can verify by checking #37 and finding if it is painful. If so, treat the kidneys.

If you find in your explorations a sore spot and do not know its name or number as listed, treat it anyway. It is calling for help. If a contact point is located where you cannot reach it, you may have to enlist the help of a friend.

You may use the tip of your index finger, your third finger, or for even more strength, reinforce your index finger by placing the third finger on top of the index finger or use the two fingertips side by side. At some points, such as #10M or #17, it is much easier to use the tip of your thumb.

Once you learn the energy centers of the body and contact any one of them which is sore or painful, give a small, fast circular movement with the index and mid-fingers before going further. This is a massage movement.

Each family should have health information for emergency purposes if a doctor is not available, or until he is available. The heart treatment is worth many, many times the price of this book alone.

Remember that each individual is different. The charts picture a contact point in a certain location, but because you may be taller, or wider or differently built, your contact point may be slightly different in location. This is really not a problem. Even if you do not know its name or what it represents, treat a sore spot; the tenderness indicates an energy leak which needs to be corrected.

The problems or disturbances you wish to treat are listed alphabetically in the index with the numbers of their contact points.

How Often to Treat

Always use only the amount of pressure you can tolerate. Pressure on contacts should be firm but not hard enough to be acutely painful. Remember, you cannot overtreat. The longer and the more often, the better. In all severe, acute or chronic conditions, treat daily for the first week; then two or three times weekly; finally once weekly. This is determined by your own needs. Sometimes much time is necessary; other times a condition will respond so fast as to be unbelievable. When the tenderness is gone, you will know that the congestion has been relieved.

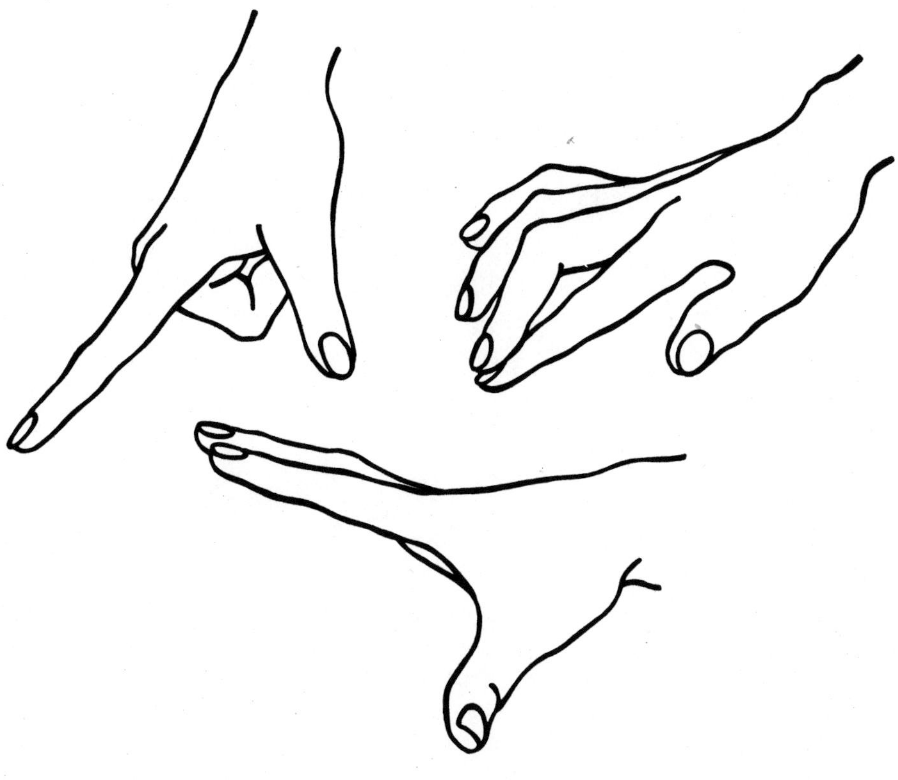

The Head
and its Pressure Points

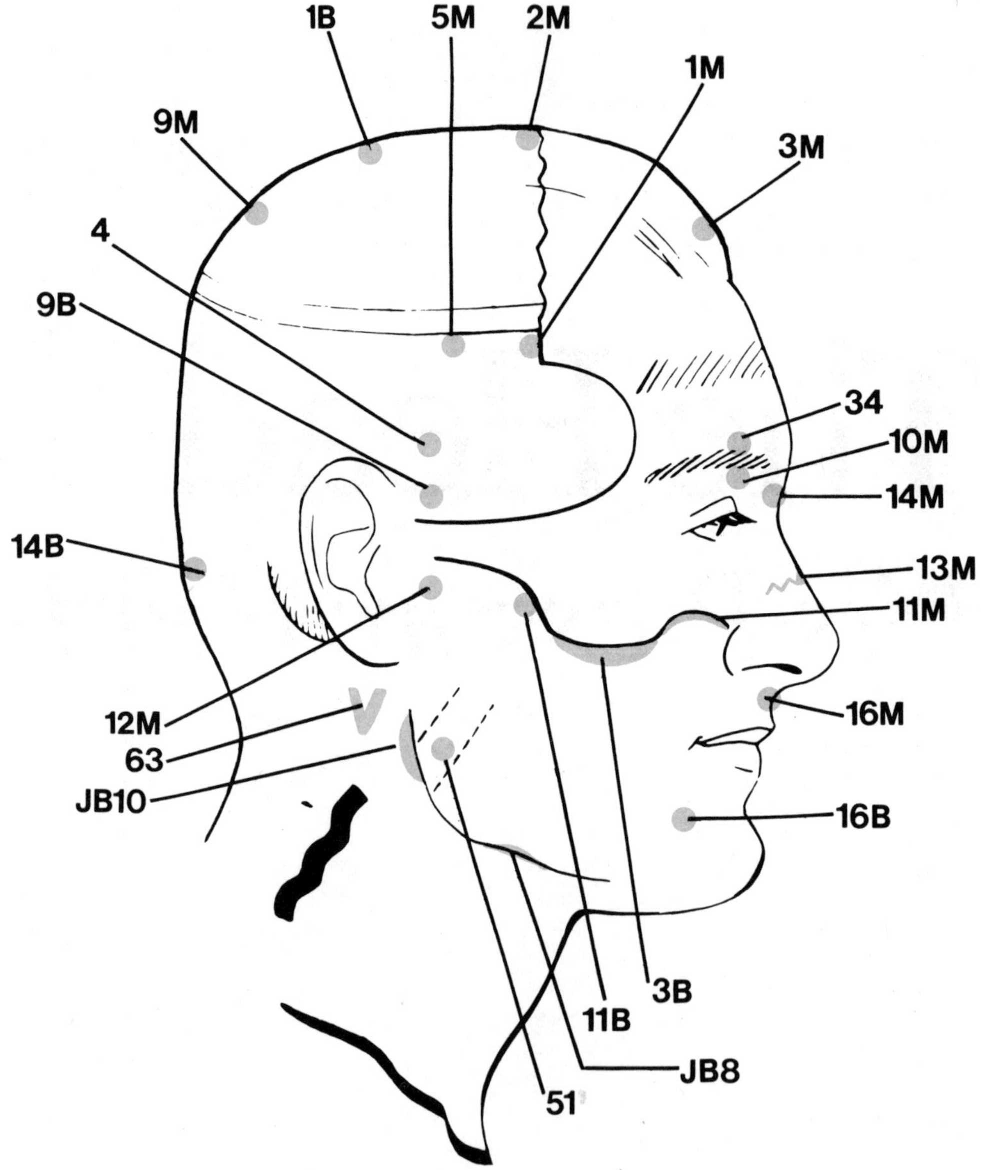
1B
5M
2M
1M
9M
3M
4
9B
34
10M
14M
14B
13M
11M
12M
63
JB10
16M
16B
3B
11B
JB8
51

Points of the Head

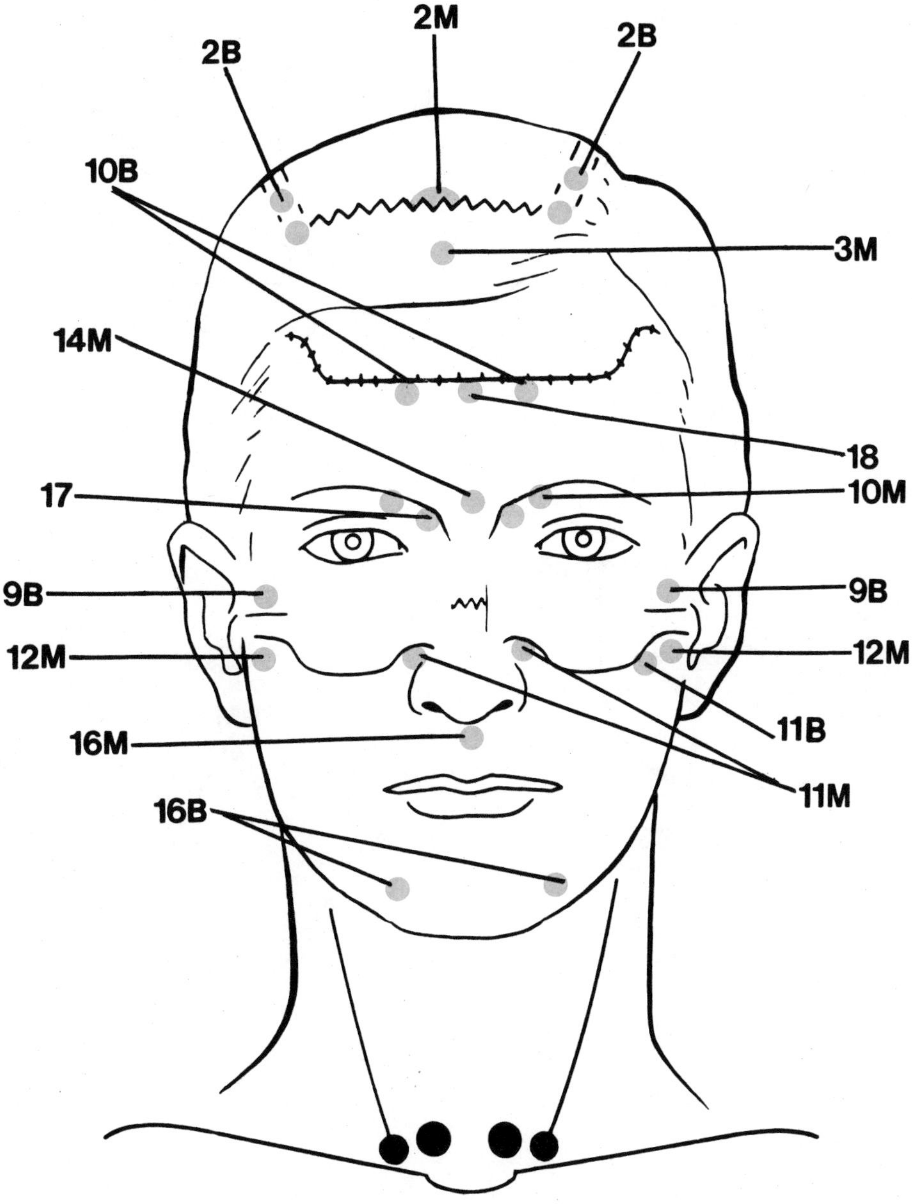

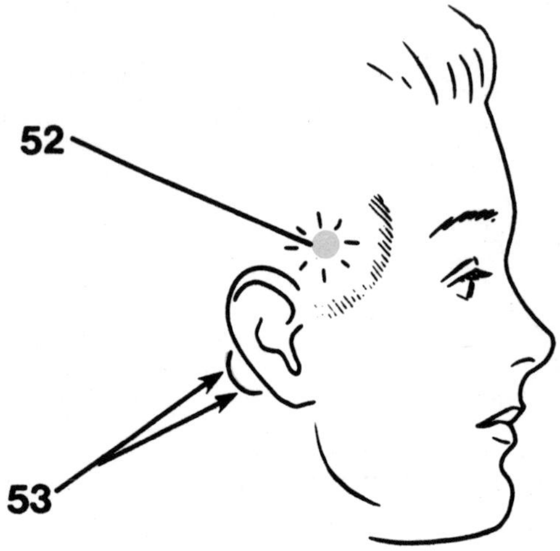
52
53

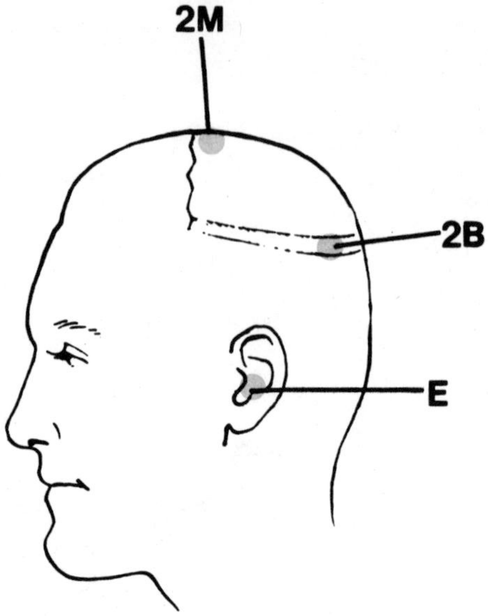
2M
2B
E

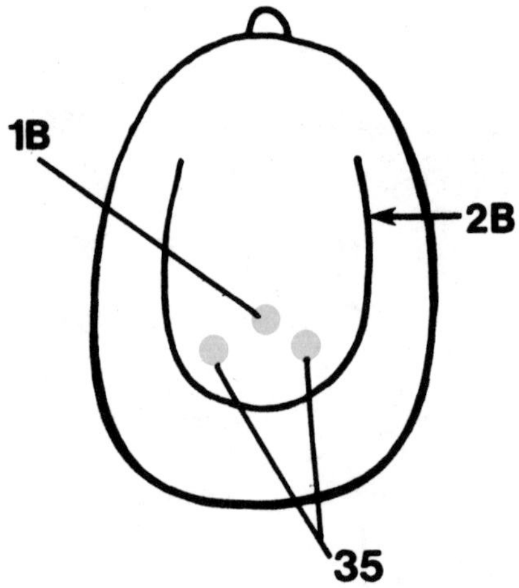
1B
2B
35

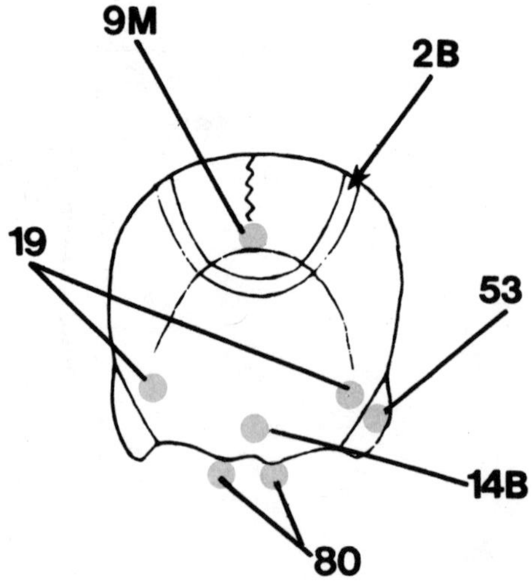
9M
2B
19
53
14B
80

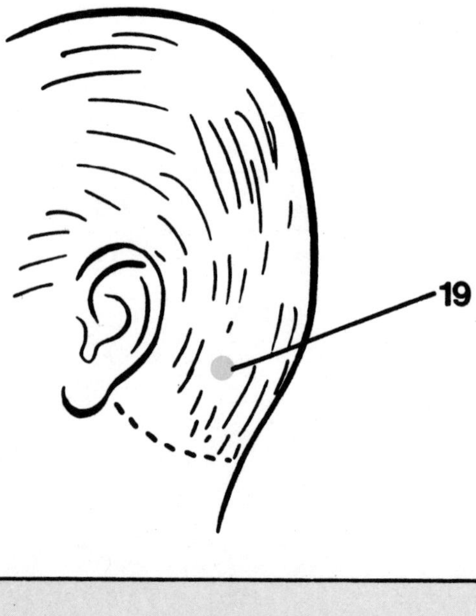
19

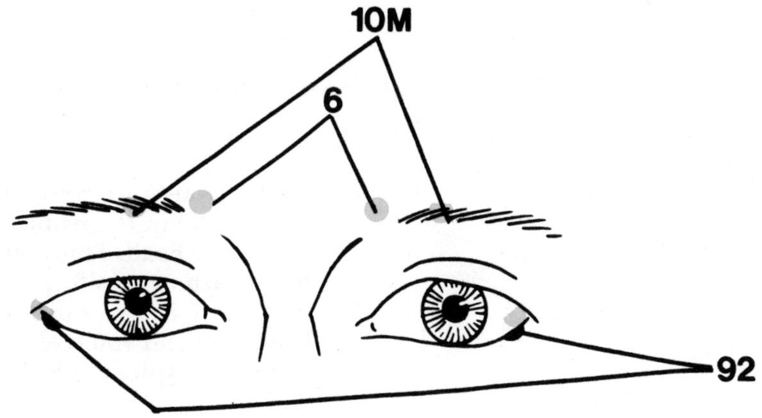

10M
6
92

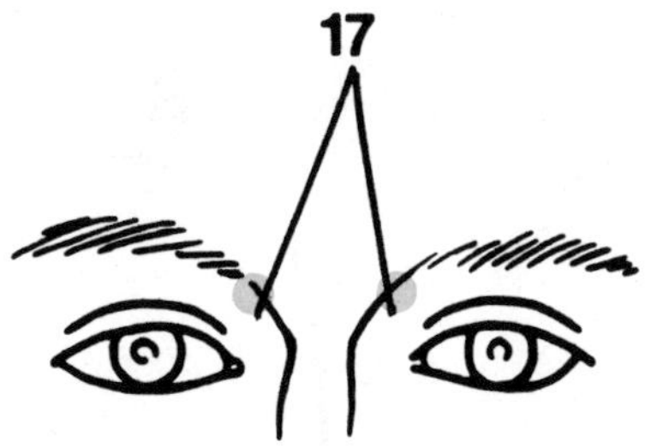

17

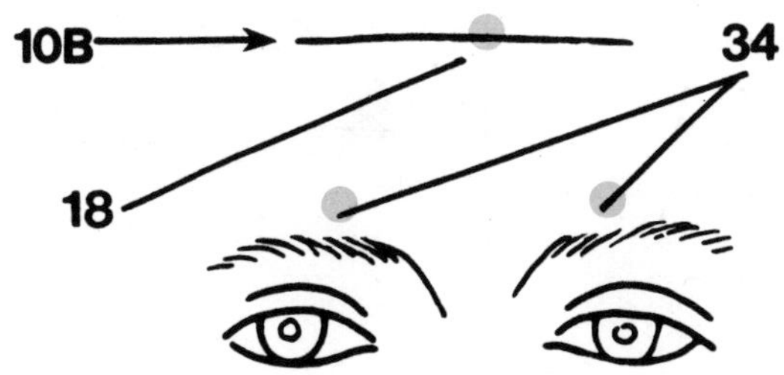

10B
34
18

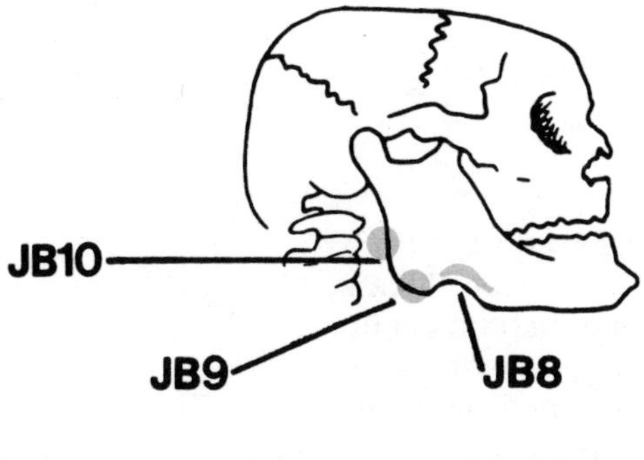

JB10
JB9
JB8

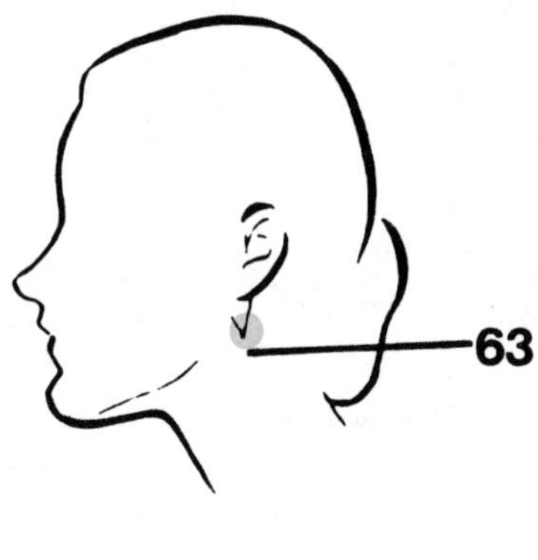

63

2M ANTERIOR FONTANELLE
pressure headache

Directly on the anterior fontanelle (soft spot) in the front part of the top of the head. This contact has to do with controlling the cranial fluid. If you have a pressure headache and you feels as if your head will explode, then the 2M will, in nearly every case, help.

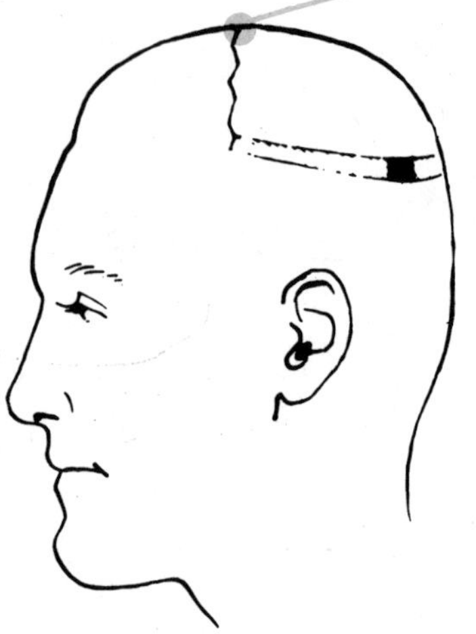

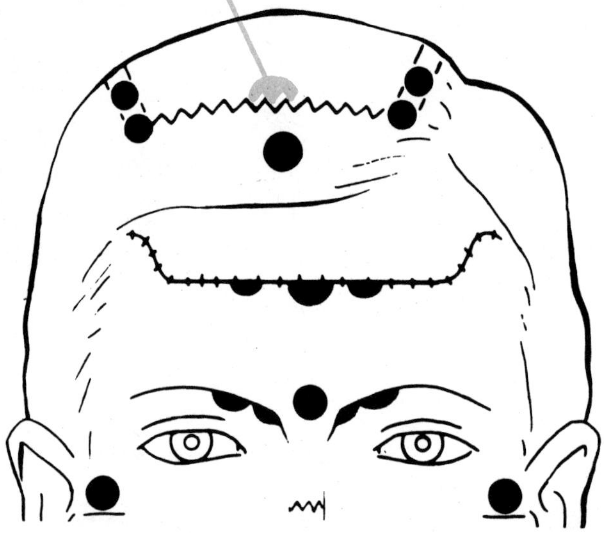

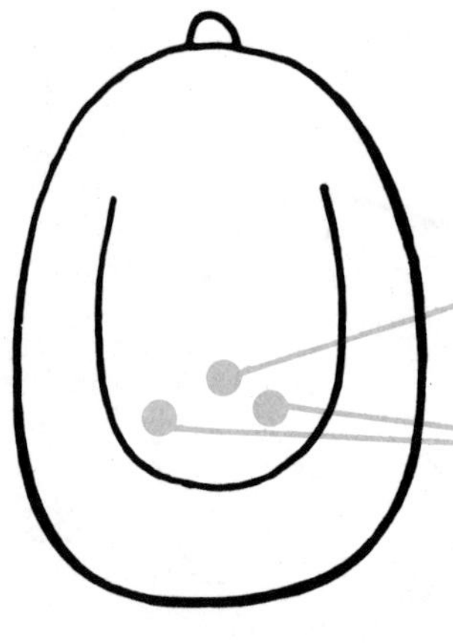

35 ***Systemic***
cerebellum

These two centers treat certain types of eye pain. They are located approximately one inch on each side of the 1B and one inch posterior. With 1B they resemble a pyramid on the head.

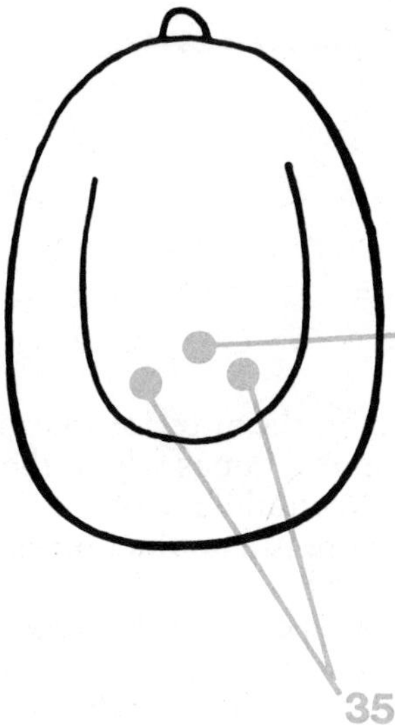

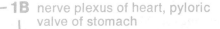

1B nerve plexus of heart, pyloric valve of stomach

Located in center top of the crown of the head, approximately one inch anterior or in front of the posterior fontanelle or soft spot. This contact goes to the pylorus or bottom valve of the stomach and also the central nerve plexus of the heart. It is also used for abdominal cramps, gas and indigestion. Some people feel the effects of this treatment all down through the body, from head to feet, as a tingling sensation.

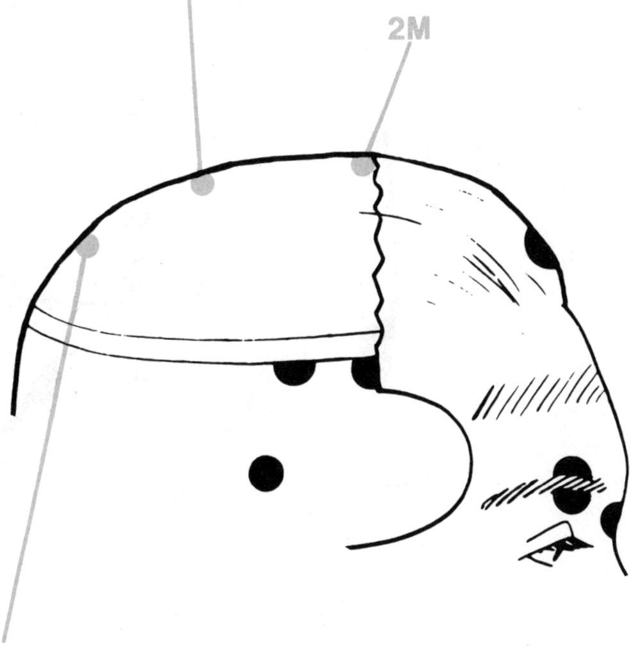

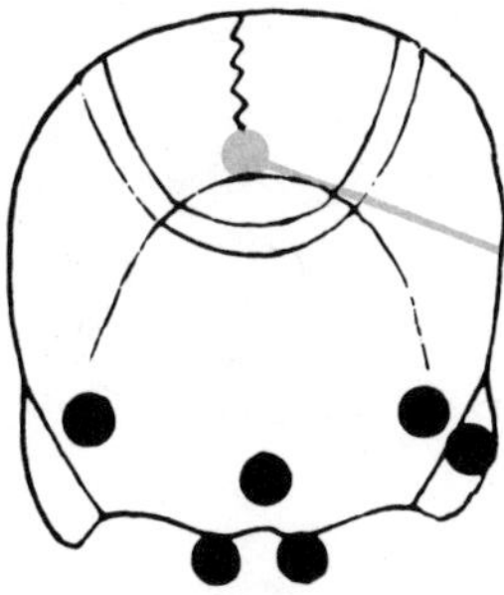

9M POSTERIOR FONTANELLE
brain, energy, bloat

Located on the posterior fontanelle and balances the energy between the pituitary and the pineal glands. Thence the energy travels down the spinal cord. It treats the brain, colon, enlarged legs, bloat and excess fluid. Very important.

5M emotional center of the brain

Just below but touching the sylvian fissure (#2B) where the parietal bones meet the frontal bone on each side of the head. The 5M's treat the emotional center of the brain. The treatment usually helps relax one, and relieves some headaches. It is to be used under a doctor's supervision only.

1M double vision, intestines

Located on the anterior margin of the temporal bones where they join the frontal bone of the forehead. There is a contact on each side of the head. Tenderness or pain on this contact denotes trouble in cranial nerves. This is where we treat the condition called diplopia, or double vision. It is also the brain contact to the intestines.

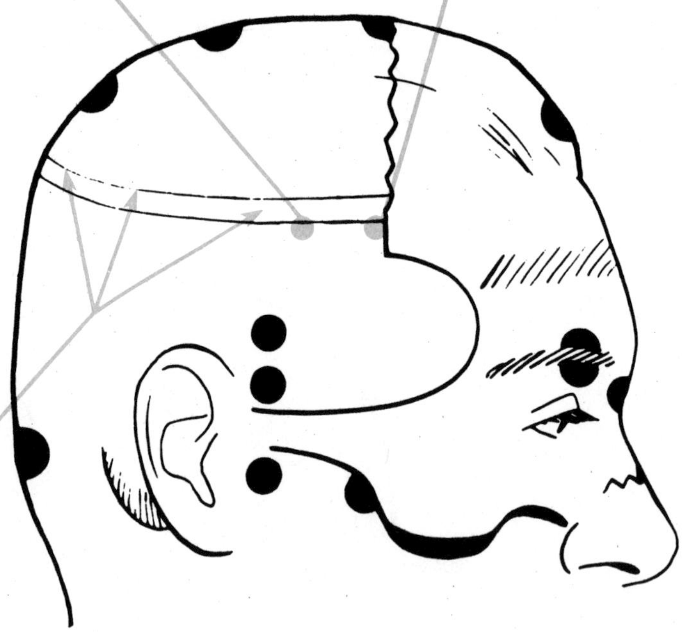

2B SYLVIAN FISSURE
capillary system, coronary arteries

A bony, horseshoe-shaped shelf called the sylvian fissure. Anywhere we touch along the crest of this contact treats some part of the capillary system. The area above and posterior to the left ear treats the coronary arteries of the heart and also all capillaries of the lungs. The anterior point treats the eyes and vocal cords. A most important contact.

3M dizziness, stomach, trachea

Located on the anterior medial line of the head approximately two inches in front of the anterior fontanelle. This contact treats the stomach, trachea and pons of the brain which has to do with the absorption of oxygen from the blood into the brain. Check first on this contact to relieve dizziness.

18 pituitary

The main head contact to the pituitary gland. Located against the underside of the 10B in the very center of the forehead. The pituitary plays a master role in the entire chemistry of the body. When this gland is congested, the pain is most severe. Press contacts #18 and #21 (see page 69) simultaneously.

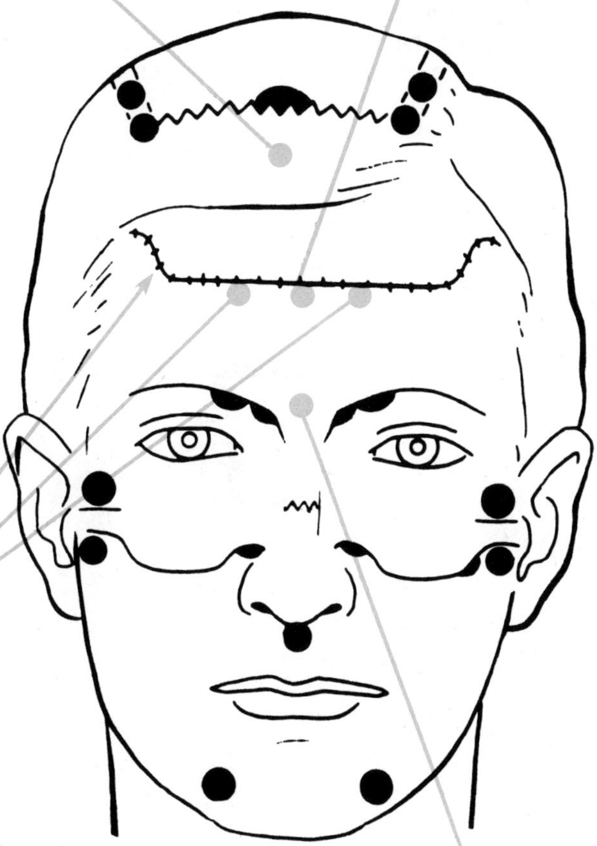

10B ***Systemic***
eyes, mental conditions

A single bony protuberance that extends from temple to temple across the center of the frontal bone and then upward for about two inches following the area just in front of the temporal junction with the frontal bone. This two-inch area affects certain eye conditions. The center part across the forehead is systemic and mental, except for two small contacts located on the bone (#10B) directly above the beginning of each eyebrow. These two contacts treat "blurred vision."

14M eyes, legs, stomach

The area between the eyebrows at the root of the nose. This is the pineal contact and is associated with such conditions as eye problems, stomach and lower leg dysfunctions.

6 brain, sinus

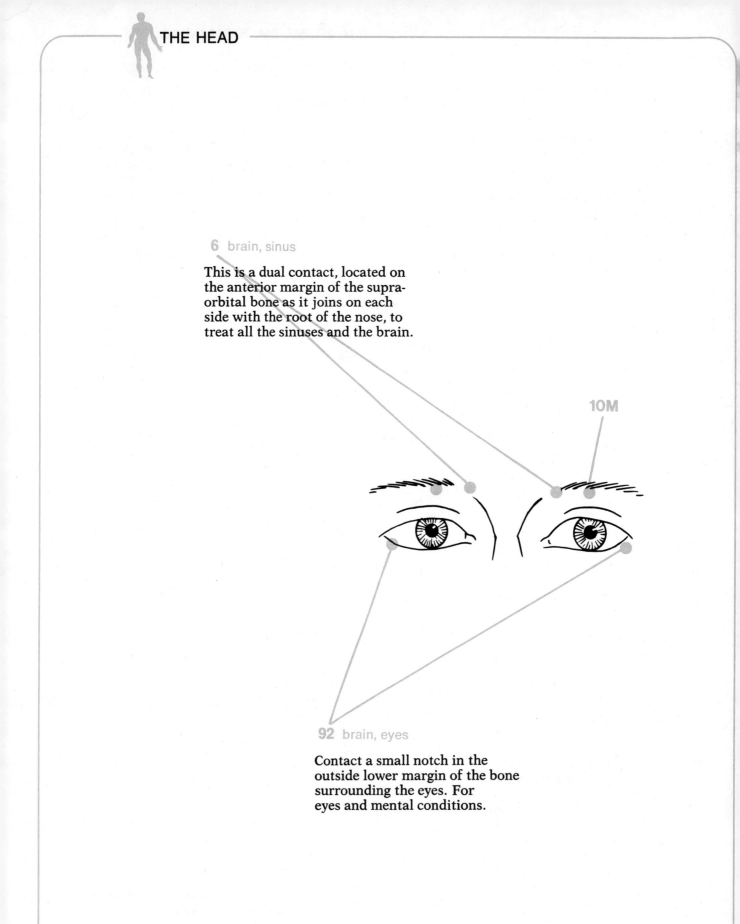

This is a dual contact, located on the anterior margin of the supra-orbital bone as it joins on each side with the root of the nose, to treat all the sinuses and the brain.

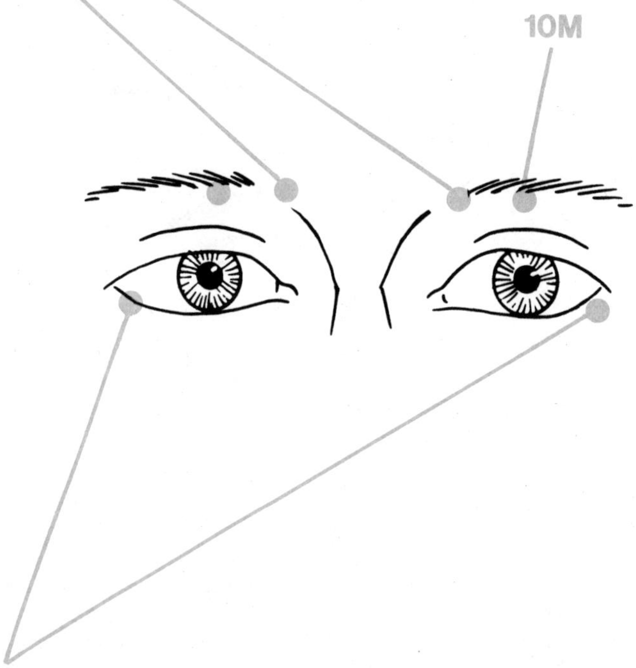

92 brain, eyes

Contact a small notch in the outside lower margin of the bone surrounding the eyes. For eyes and mental conditions.

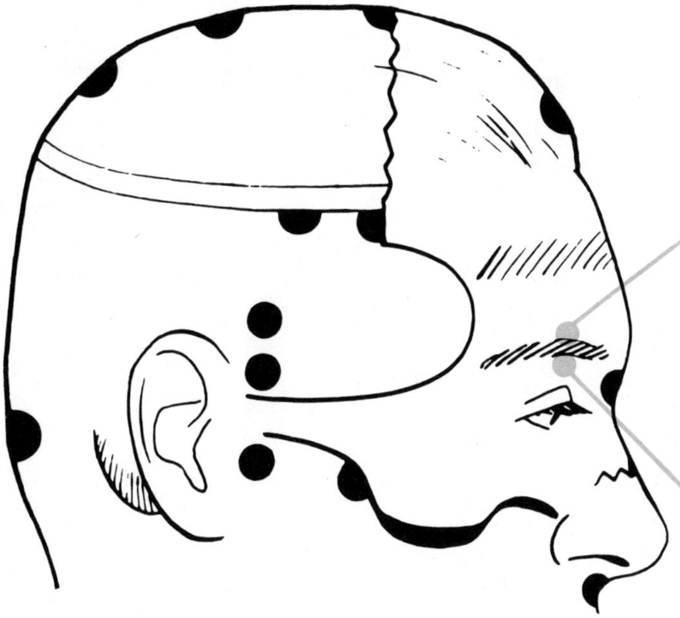

34 brain, energy, food poisoning

Treats the eyes, the frontal lobe of the brain and affects the consciousness and intestines. These two contacts are located directly above the center of the eyebrows against the frontal bone of the forehead. Also for food poisoning. If you become sleepy while driving,press #34's for a few minutes.

10M ***Systemic***
brain, gallbladder, liver, pleurisy, sciatica

These are dual and located in the supraorbital notch beneath each eyebrow. Contact with the tip of your thumbs to treat the frontal brain and the covering of both lungs (pleura). They are the brain contacts to liver, gall bladder and even treat a type of sciatic pain in hip and legs. Very important.

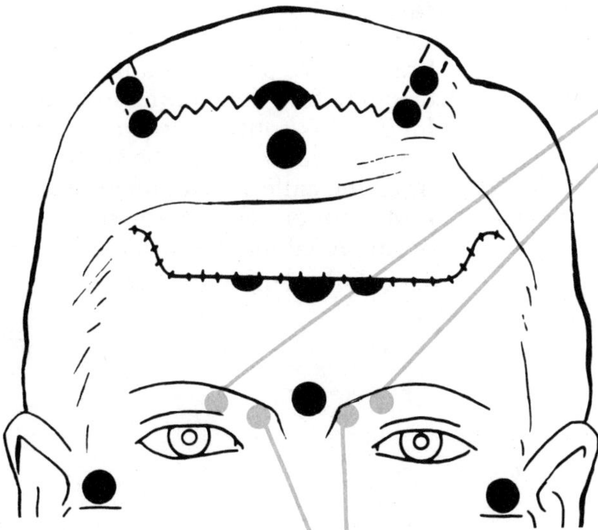

17 eyestrain, stomach

The contact for eyestrain. Locate contact #6's on either side of the bridge of the nose. Then, using the tip of the thumb, slide straight back under the eyebrows and press upward. Any painful area found in this location can be treated with your thumb. Eyestrain is one of the most common causes of headaches. Number 17 is also a treating point for the stomach.

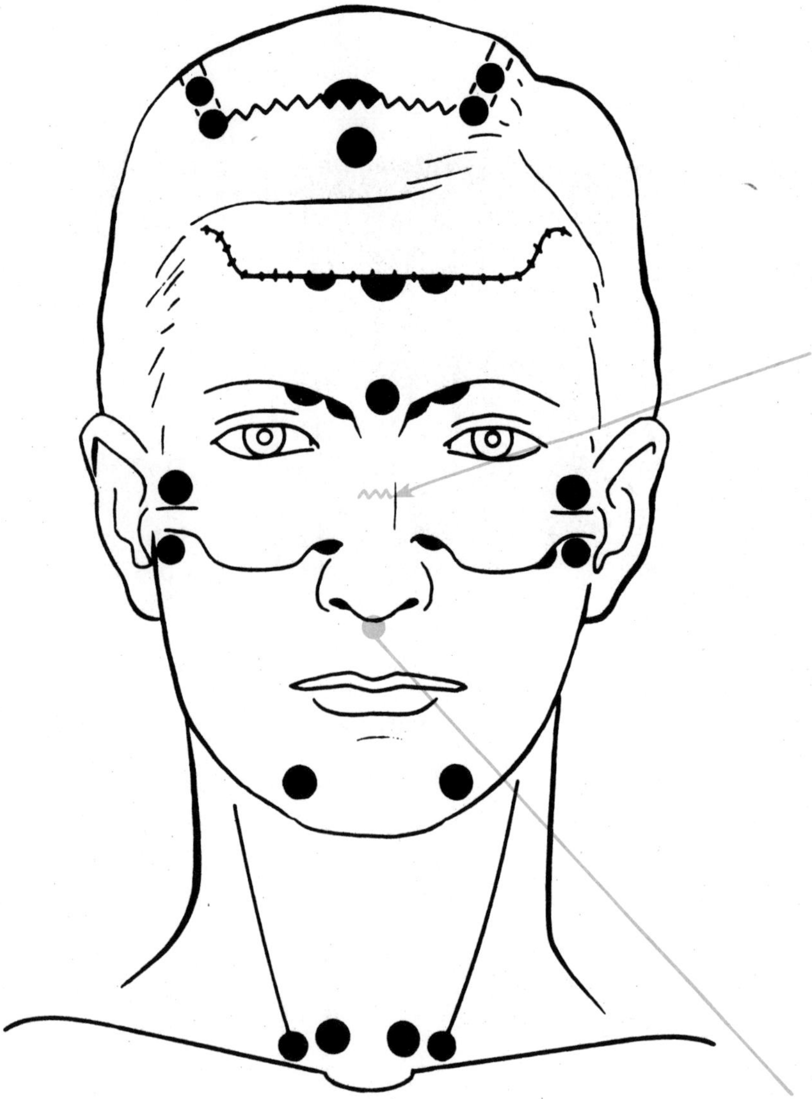

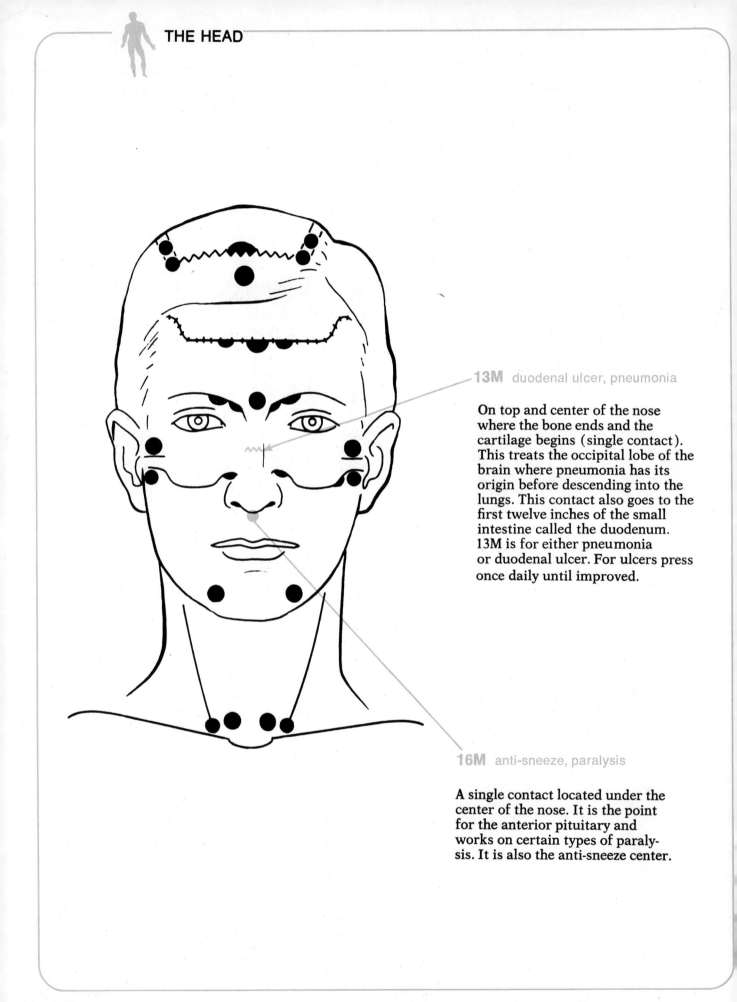

13M duodenal ulcer, pneumonia

On top and center of the nose where the bone ends and the cartilage begins (single contact). This treats the occipital lobe of the brain where pneumonia has its origin before descending into the lungs. This contact also goes to the first twelve inches of the small intestine called the duodenum. 13M is for either pneumonia or duodenal ulcer. For ulcers press once daily until improved.

16M anti-sneeze, paralysis

A single contact located under the center of the nose. It is the point for the anterior pituitary and works on certain types of paralysis. It is also the anti-sneeze center.

4 brain, spinal nerves

These two contacts are located approximately two inches above the 12M contacts and have to do with the brain and the spinal nerves.

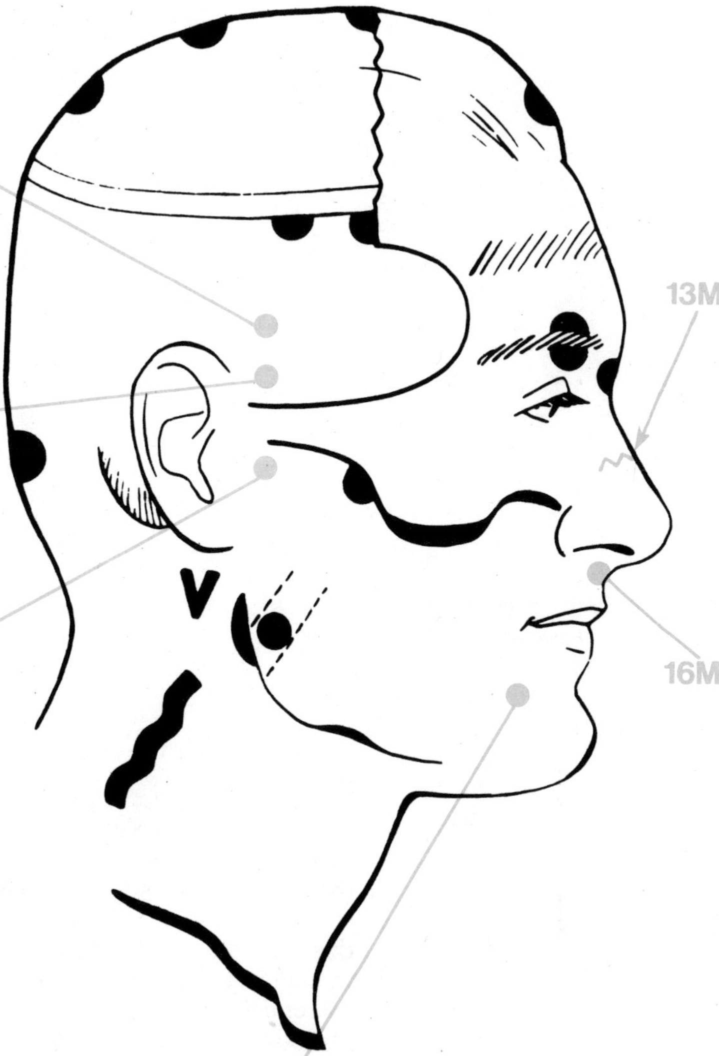

9B colon, kidneys

These are dual and are located at the superior distal end of the cheekbones just in front of each ear. They are the brain contacts to the kidneys and colon.

12M arteriosclerosis, heart, muscles, veins

Located against the hinge of each jawbone, just below #9B, and touching the front of the ear. Treatment here is for arteriosclerosis, heart and body muscles, the eustachian tubes, veins of lungs, eyes and body, heart valves and certain types of heart attacks. *Note*: In heart problems where these are painful, press both contacts simultaneously.

16B head colds, posterior pituitary

Located directly below the outer corners of the lips, this is on each side of the chin at the center of the lower jawbone on the mental foramen. It has to do with the posterior pituitary and is a specific treating point for head colds.

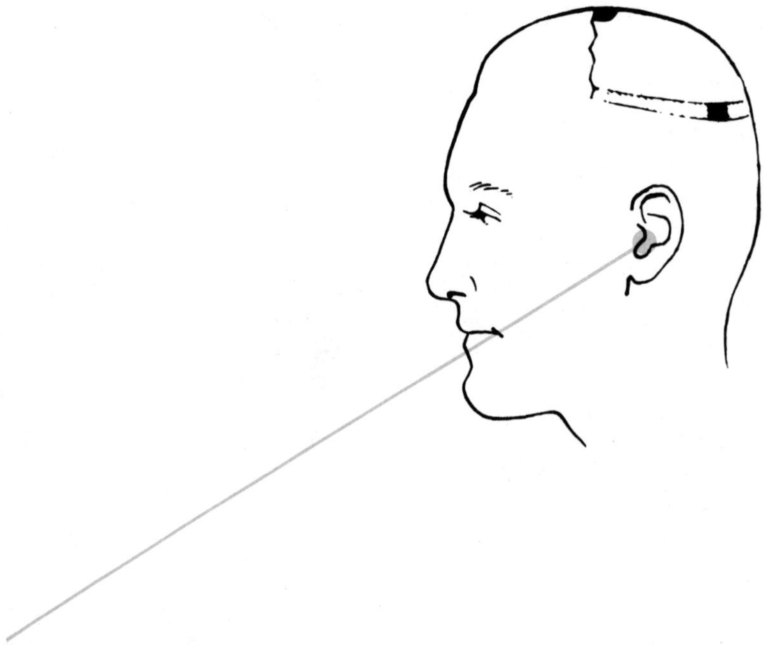

E blood pressure

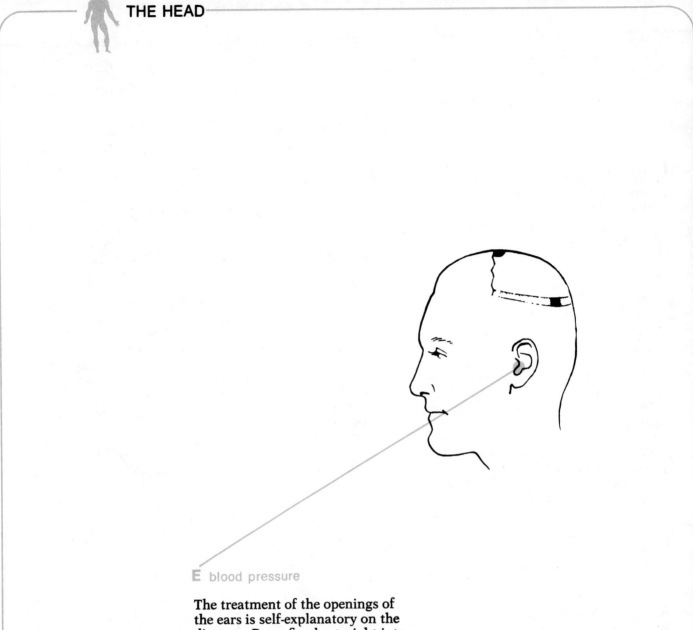

The treatment of the openings of the ears is self-explanatory on the diagram. Press firmly straight into the ear, then lift slightly forward toward the nose. If it is needed, this treatment will be felt all through the body or in the extremities, and the blood pressure may be reduced at the first treatment. Hold contacts for several minutes.

11B infection

Check diagram carefully on these dual contacts, located on the posterior aspect of the cheekbones. When painful they may indicate infection somewhere in the head or body.

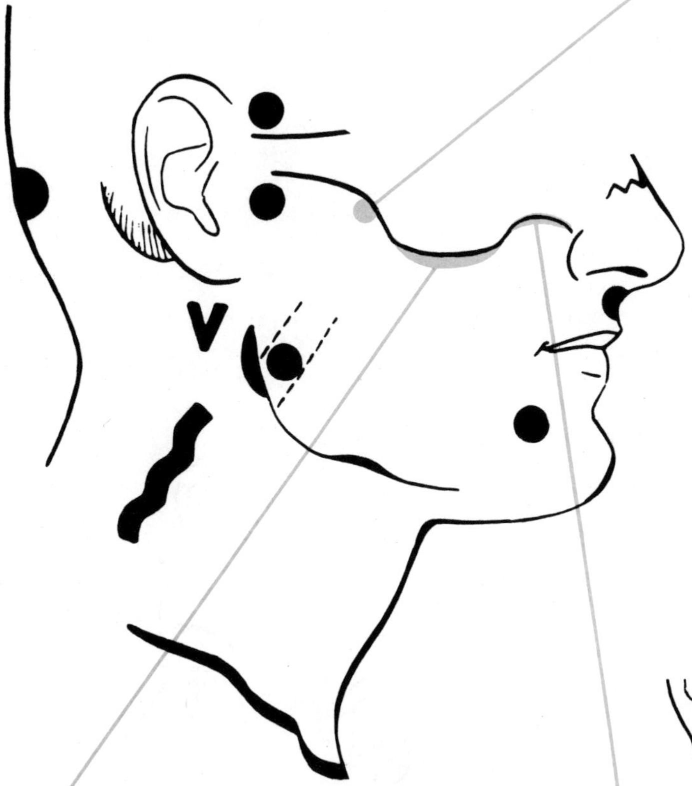

3B sinusitis

Against the inferior margin of both cheekbones. They refer to mucous membranes or lining of tissues. Check these for sinusitis.

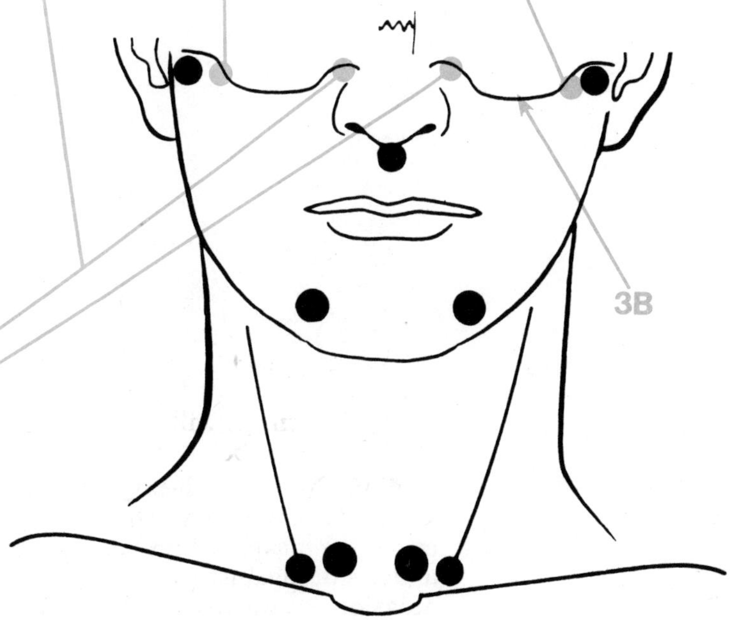

11M allergies, bronchi, lungs

Press firmly in and upward on tissue just adjoining each side of the nose. As you press upward you will touch the underside of a small, bony shelf. These are the 11M's and treat the maxillary sinuses, allergies and nasal obstructions. They are the brain contacts to the bronchial tubes and lungs.

52 abdomen, excess fluid, eyes, heart, lungs, stomach

In the very center of each temple will be found a soft spot as though there were an opening into the brain. Feel for tenderness or pain even around the center of this very small apparent opening. Contacting here treats intestines, colon and the peritoneum which is a large apron-like tissue that covers and protects the contents of the abdomen. Peritonitis is a medical term meaning infection of the peritoneum. Treat also for stomach, lungs, heart, abdominal bloat, excess fluid and the eyes.

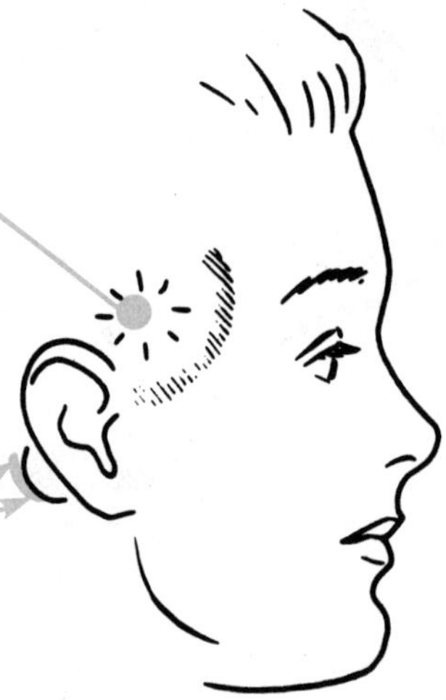

53 MASTOID
ears, intestines

Feel just behind each ear and you will find a small bone. This is called the mastoid. Press on the under side, against, and also, on occasion, a little to the side of it; it influences the intestines, colon and ears.

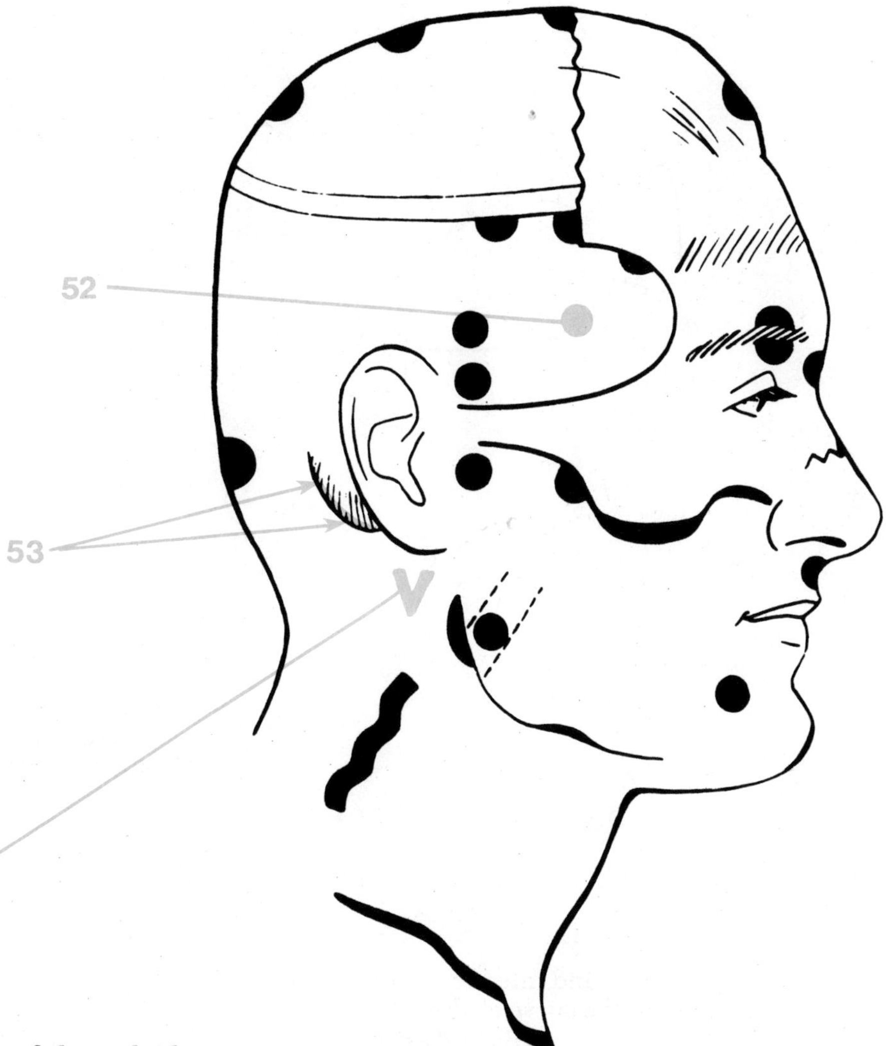

Located on the tip of the styloid—press below each ear. This contact affects the brain in certain cases. May be indicated in amnesia cases.

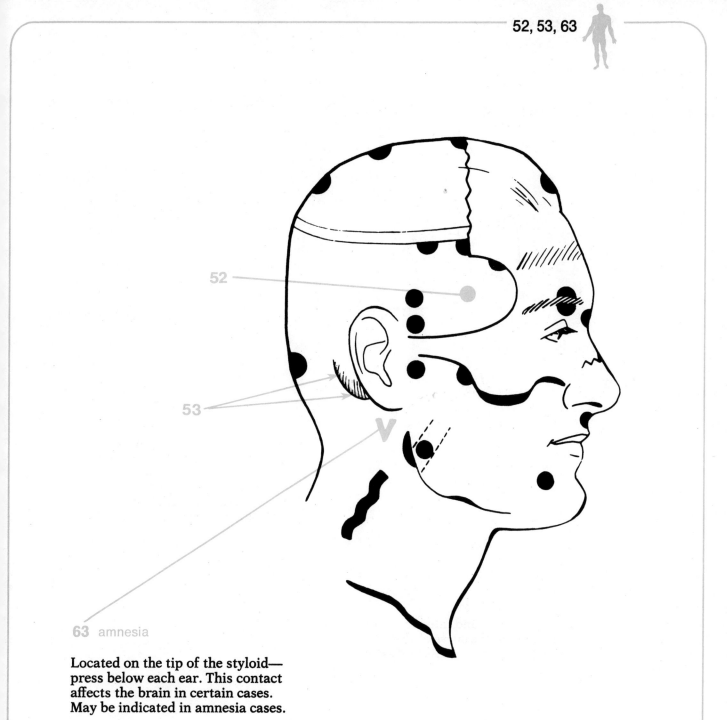

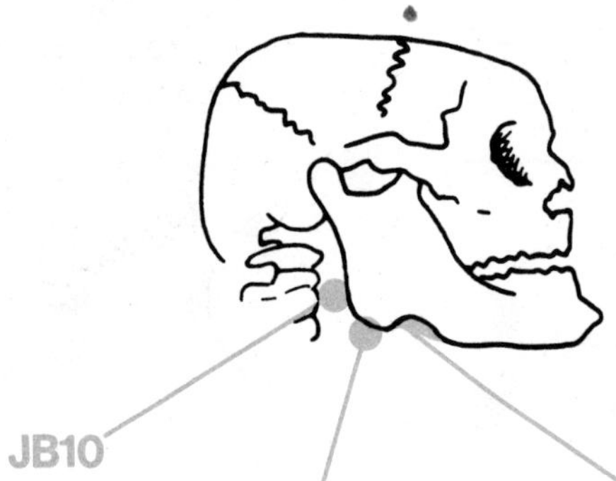

JB8 toothache

Located under each side of the lower jawbone is a notch in the bone. Feel underneath and toward the back of the underside of this bone until you feel the notch. Press for toothache.

JB9 intestines

Treats colon and intestines. It is located on the curve of the jawbone between JB8 and JB10.

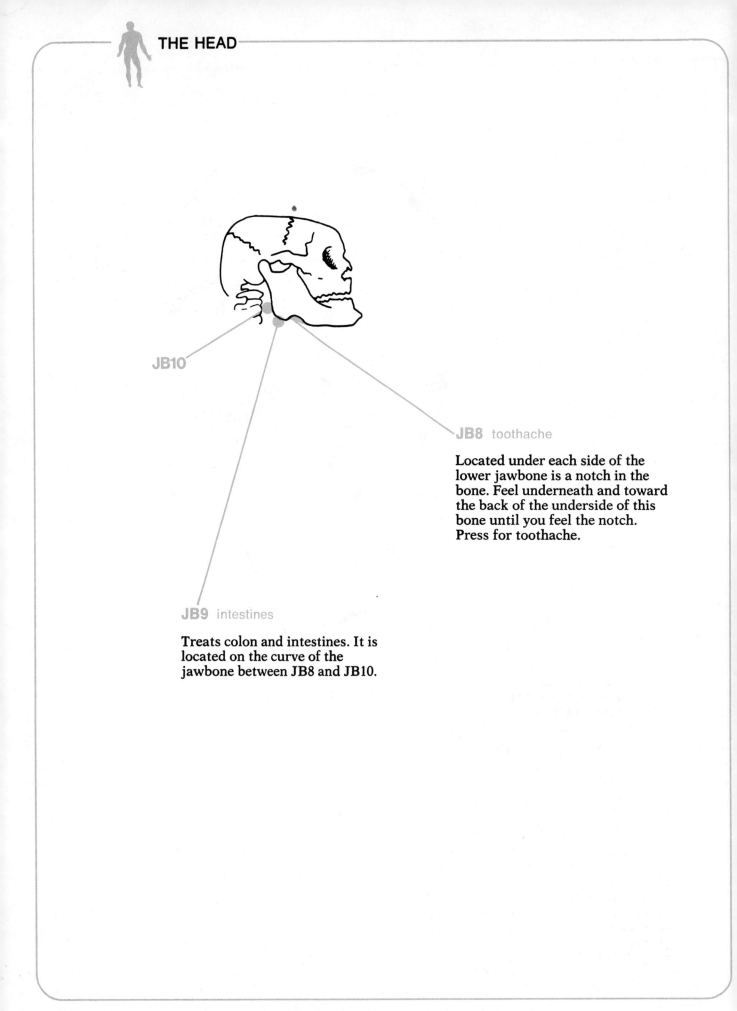

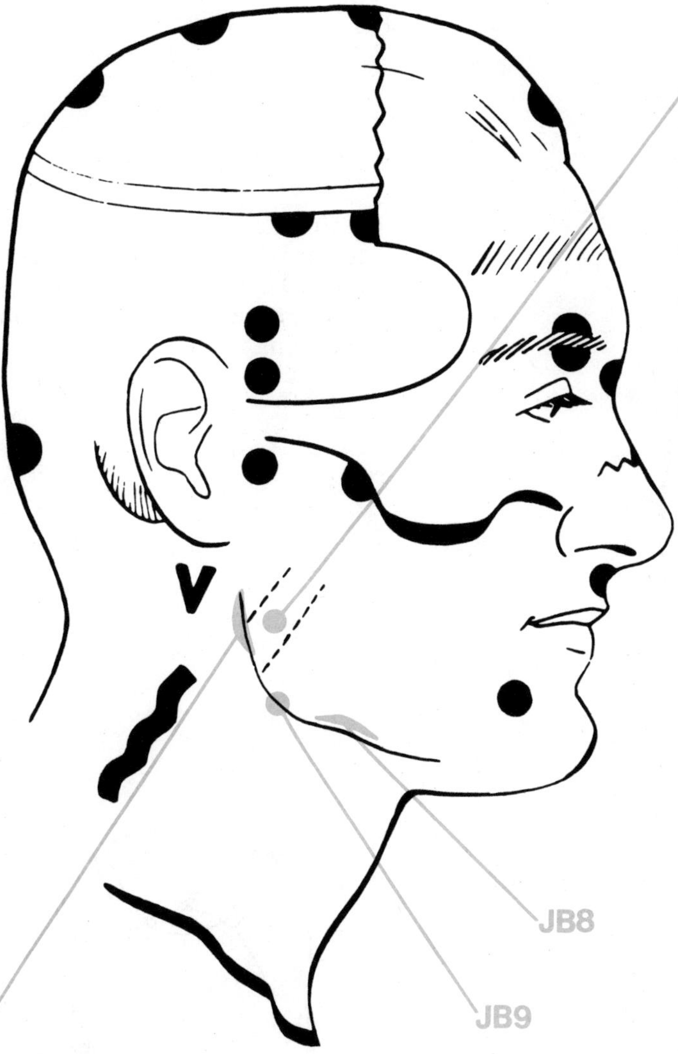

51 facial muscles, mumps

These two contacts are against the chewing or masseter muscles on the lower jawbone. Press for all the facial muscles and eyes and premature wrinkles; also for mumps, and the effects of mumps on the reproductive organs.

JB10 eyes, intoxication

Put your index finger on the posterior aspect of jawbone just under each ear and pull forward. In all cases of glaucoma, intoxication, and in people who wear or are about to get bifocal glasses, pain will be felt on these contacts. JB10 influences very strongly all the fluids going into the eyes. Treatment here will be felt as a warmth behind the eyes as circulation becomes balanced in that area. If temporarily nauseated, stop for a time then return to treating.

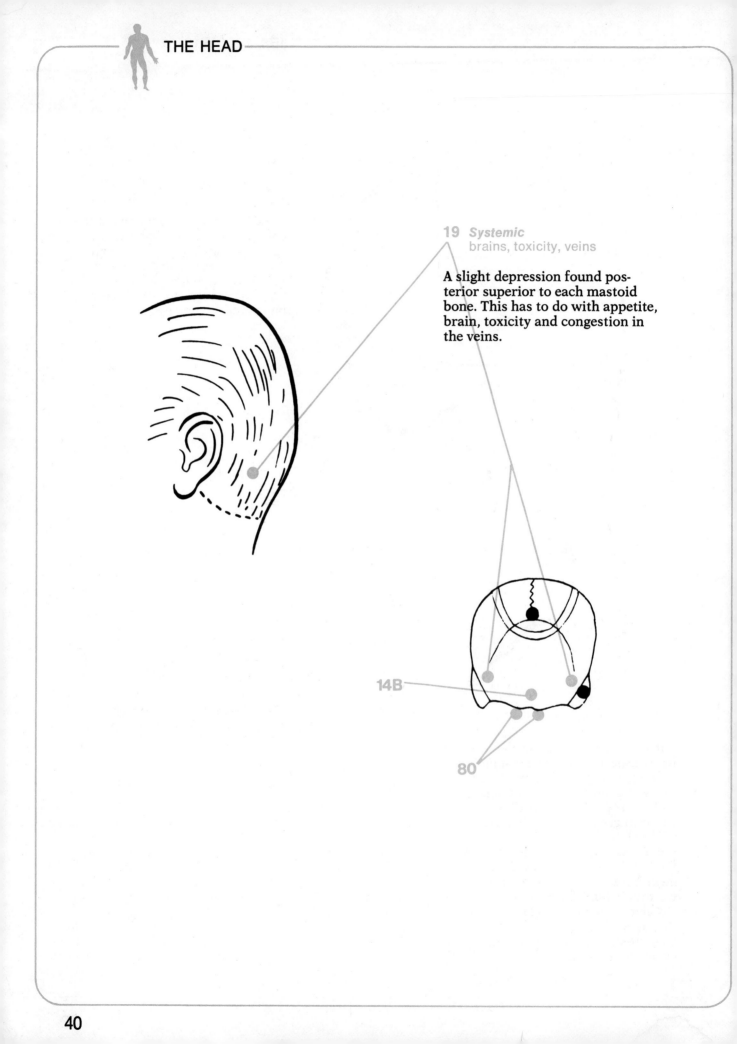

19 ***Systemic***
brains, toxicity, veins

A slight depression found posterior superior to each mastoid bone. This has to do with appetite, brain, toxicity and congestion in the veins.

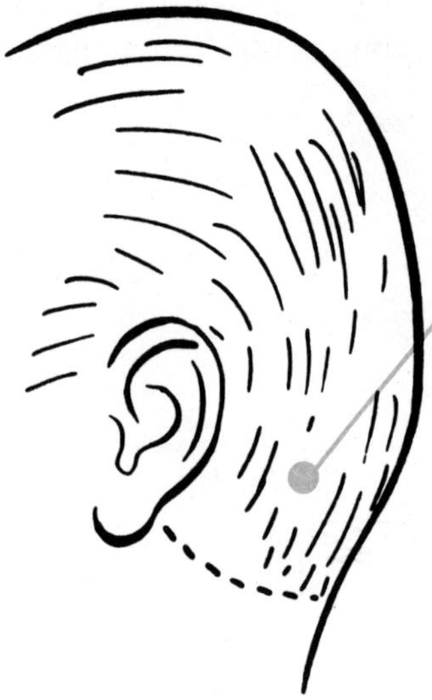

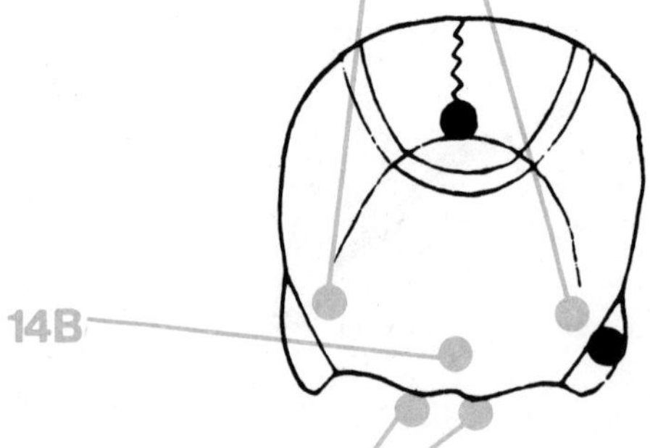

14B indigestion, stroke

The posterior inferior occipital protuberance on the under side of the back of the skull in the center. This contacts the medulla of the brain and treats stroke. It also is the brain contact to the pancreas and the first contact to think of if one has lots of gas or indigestion.

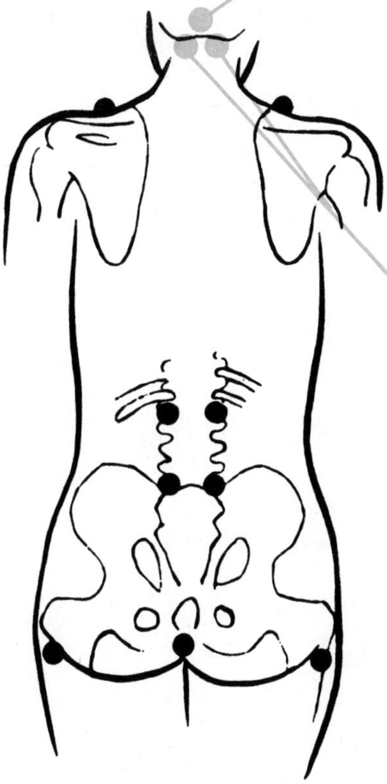

POSTERIOR ASPECT

80 head pains, nosebleeds, spleen

Located under the base of the skull on each side of center. This is the brain contact to the spleen and treats head and eye pains and nosebleeds. *Note*: Nosebleeds may indicate spleen trouble.

The Neck
and its Pressure Points

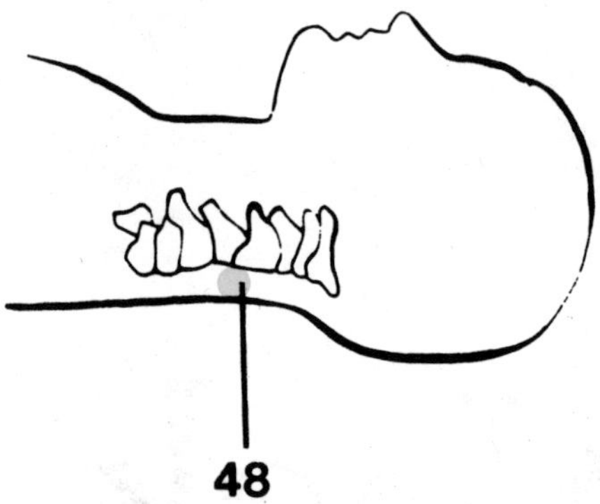
48

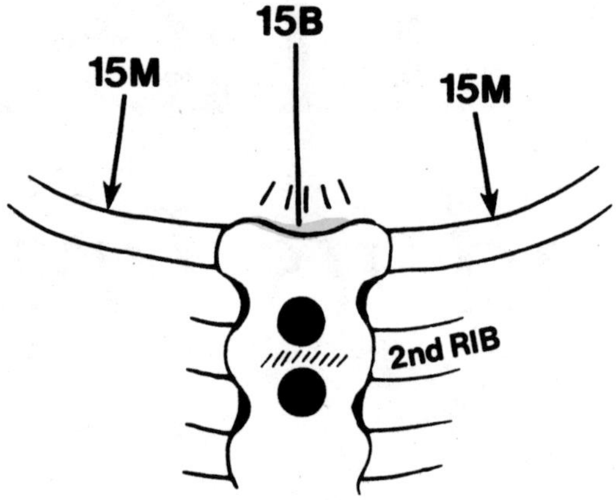
15B
15M
15M
2nd RIB

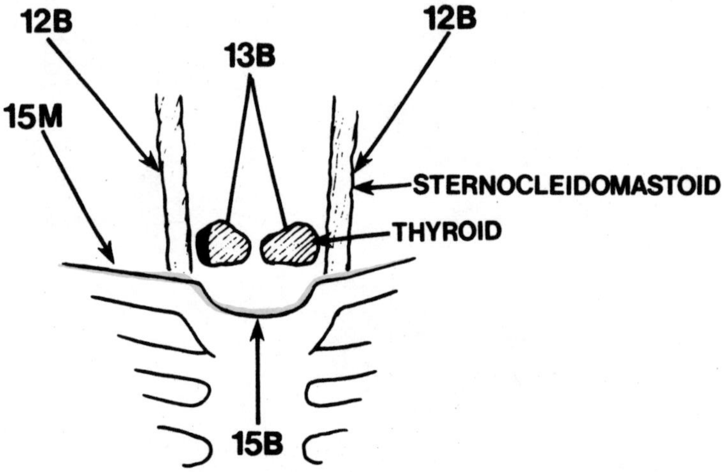
12B
12B
13B
15M
STERNOCLEIDOMASTOID
THYROID
15B

Points of the Neck

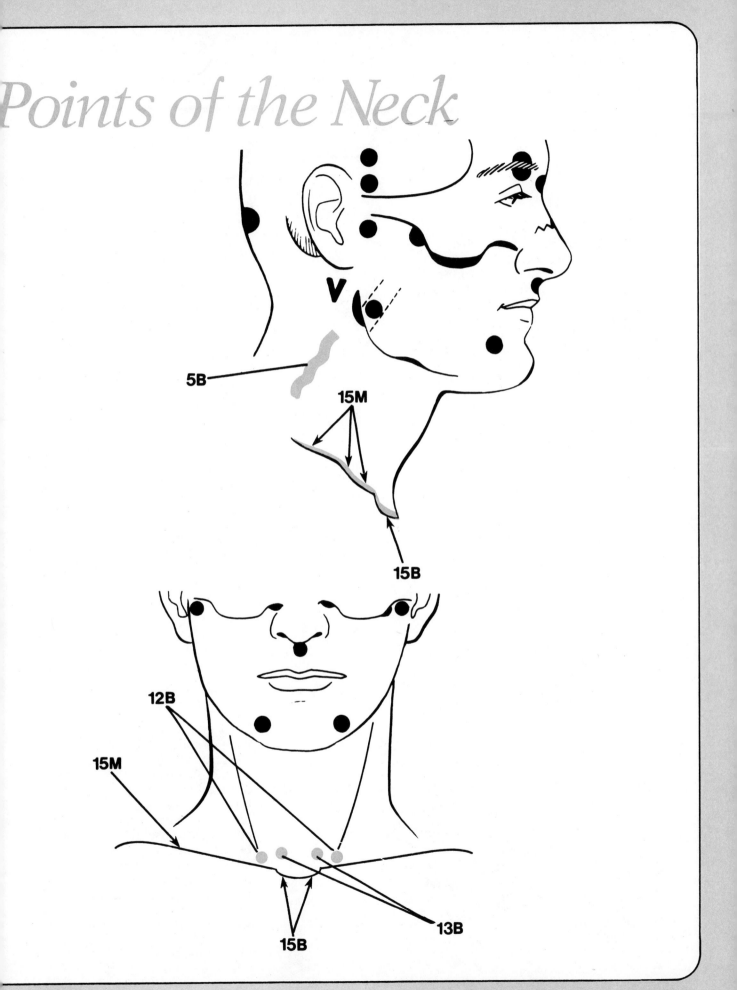

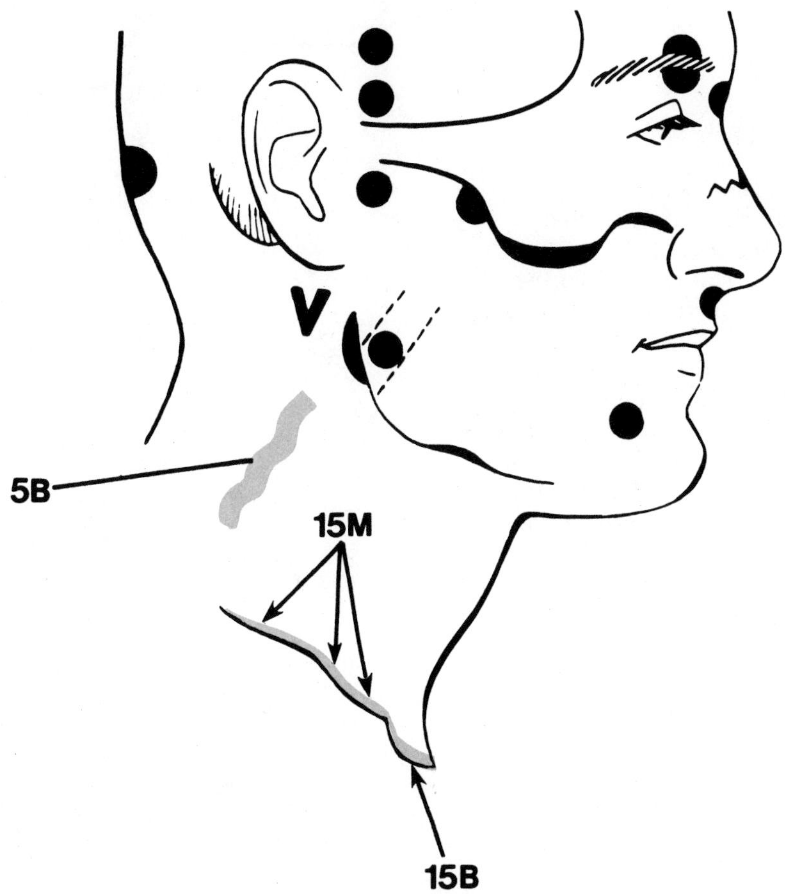

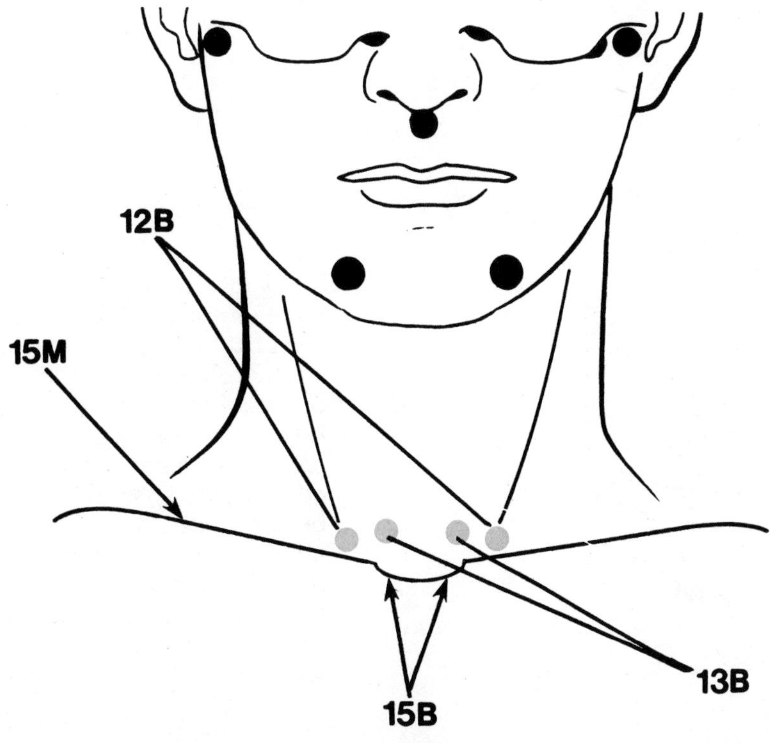

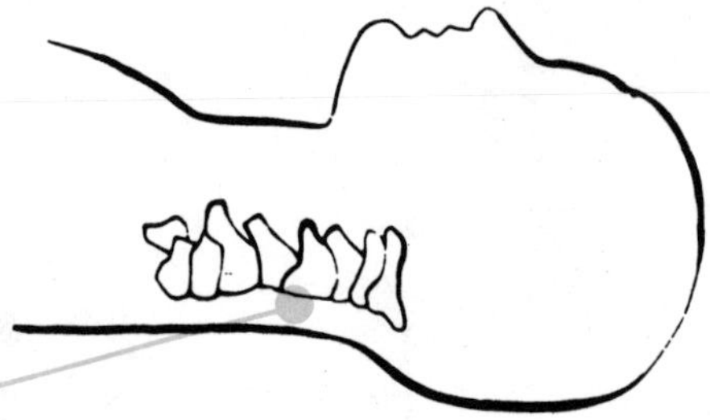

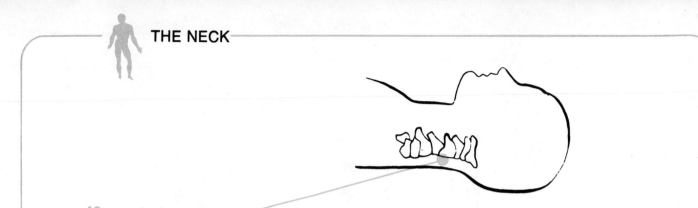

48 lymph, thoracic duct

The lymph (single contact) is located approximately at the center of the back of the neck on the third cervical spinal process. This is the vital contact to balance the electrical forces in the thoracic duct. It is the common trunk of all lymphatic vessels of the body except those on the right side of the head, neck and thorax, the right lung and right side of heart, and the convex surface of the liver. It conveys the greater part of the lymph and chyle into the blood. The thoracic duct extends upward from the 2nd lumbar vertebra to the base of the neck. This is a good one to check and press first.

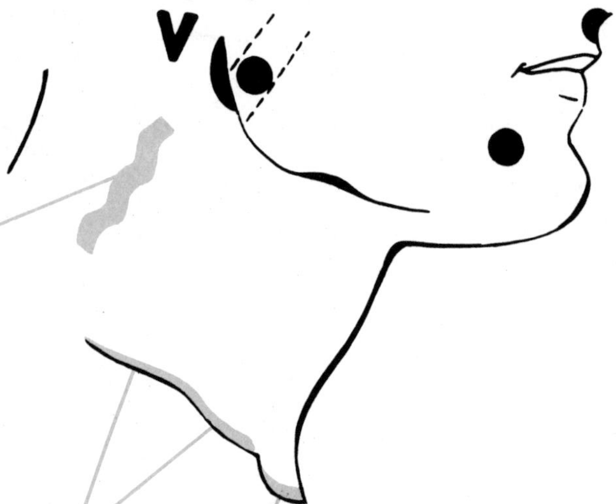

5B ***Systemic***
abdomen

Along the lateral cervical neck muscles against the transverse bony processes of the vertebrae. These points have to do with intestines, colon, appendix, etc., but care must be exercised in treatment. Press very gently!

15M

15B brain, esophagus, hernia, throat, ptosis

The superior margin of the breast-bone or sternum. Pull down on top of this bone for proper contact. This opens the top valve of the stomach, treats and helps fatten the esophagus and abdominal organs such as kidneys, uterus, etc. It is also useful in correcting hernia to lift the weight off the abdominal walls and let nature heal the hernia. It also treats the front and back of the throat. The 15B is shaped like a teacup. When we pull on the side of this cup we treat that side of the throat and up into the brain.

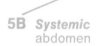

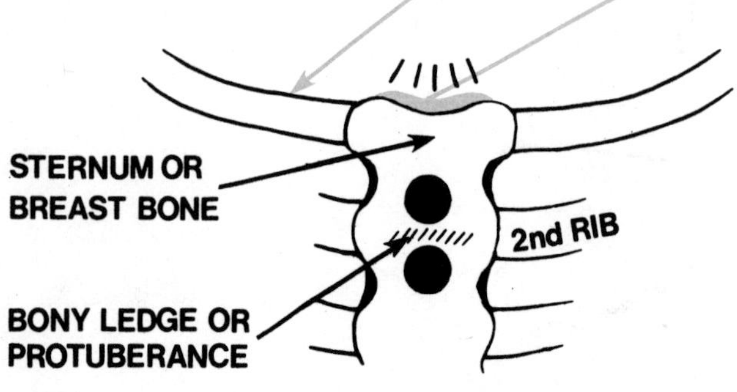

12B STERNOCLEIDOMASTOID MUSCLE
Systemic
arms, heart

One on each side of the base of the neck on the anterior lateral wall of the sternocleidomastoid muscle as it terminates in the supraclavicular fossa. Left 12B controls the left side of the heart, as in angina pectoris, and the left arm. Right side activates the right arm and right side of body.

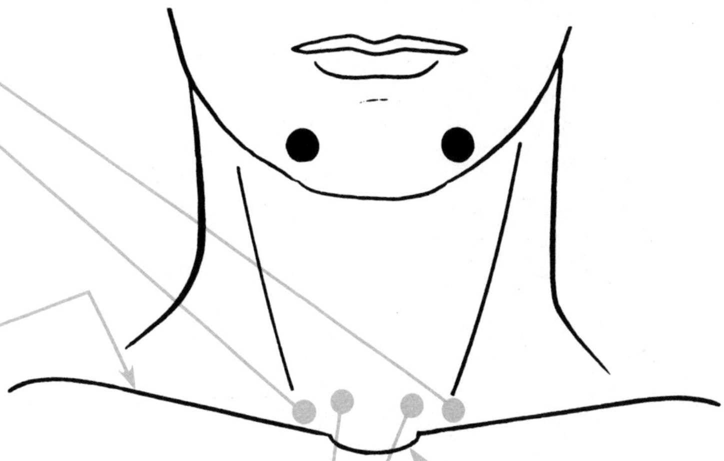

15M metabolism

The superior margin of both collarbones called the clavicle. It may influence metabolism and is very important.

13B THYROID
metabolism

A dual contact as the thyroid has two lobes. The thyroid has to do with the metabolism of the body. A malfunctioning thyroid can cause heart palpitation, loss of weight and excessive weight. It is also a factor in controlling body temperature.

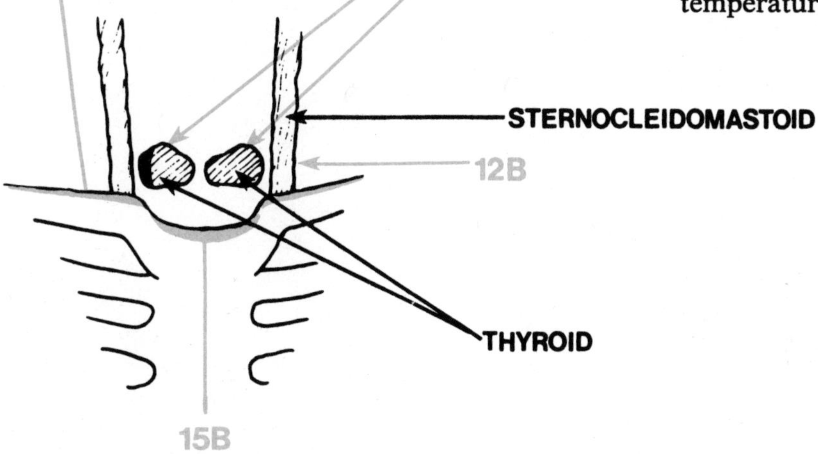

The Body

and its Pressure Points

The 40 Pressure

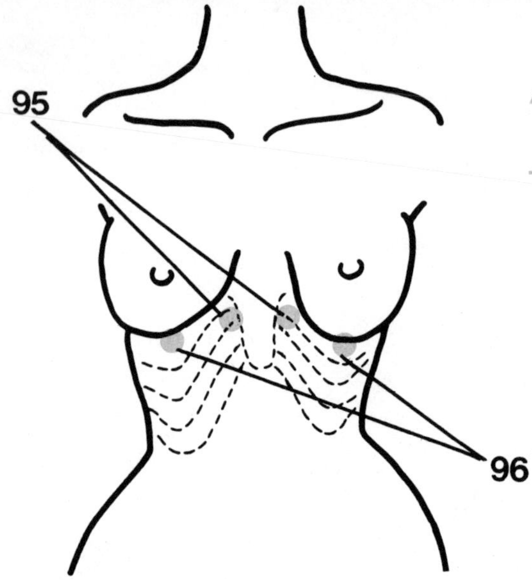

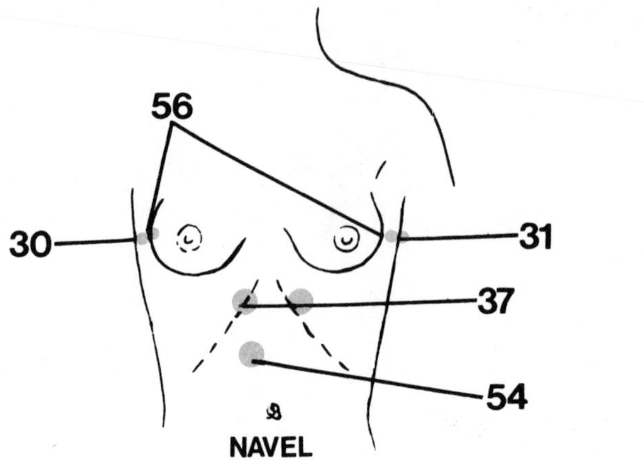

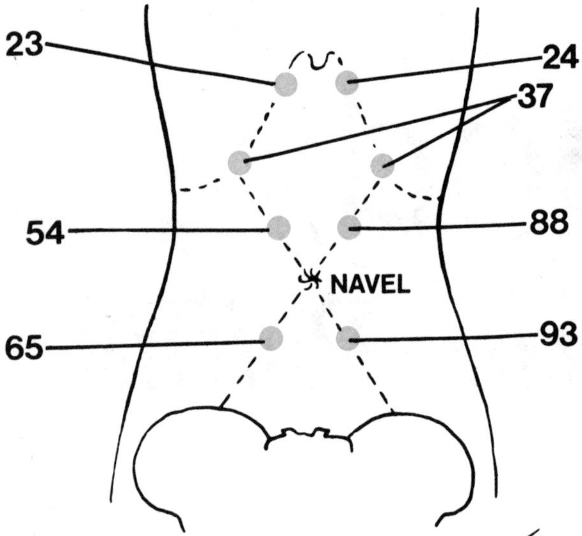

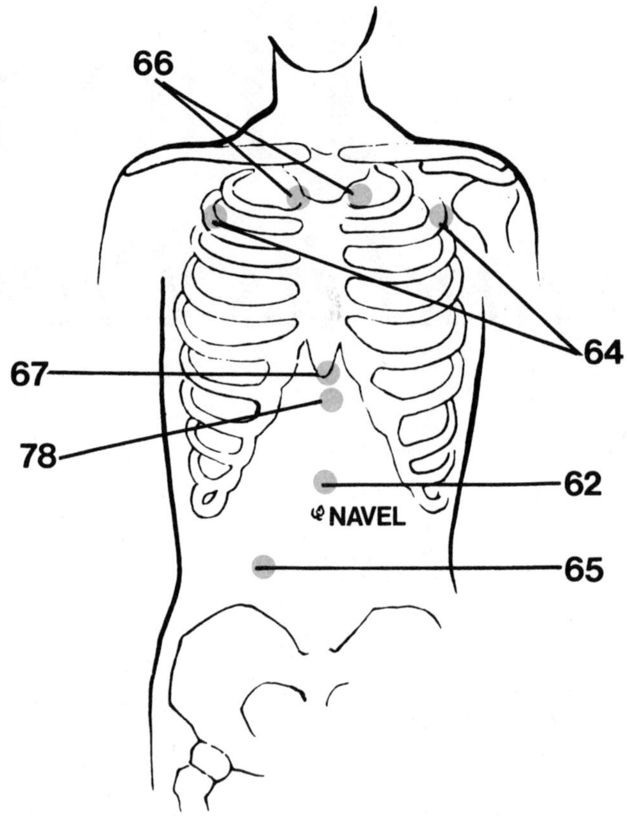

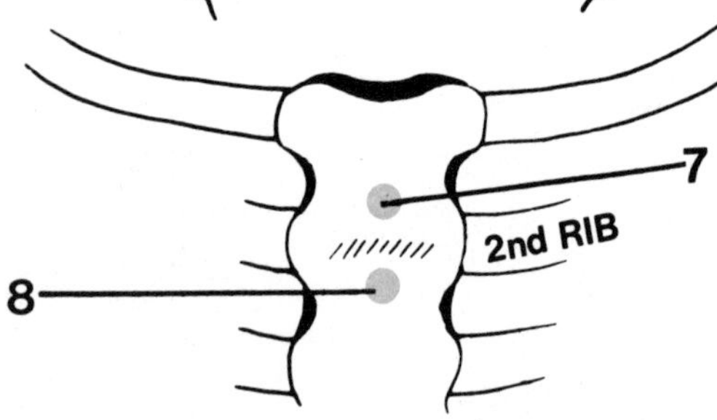

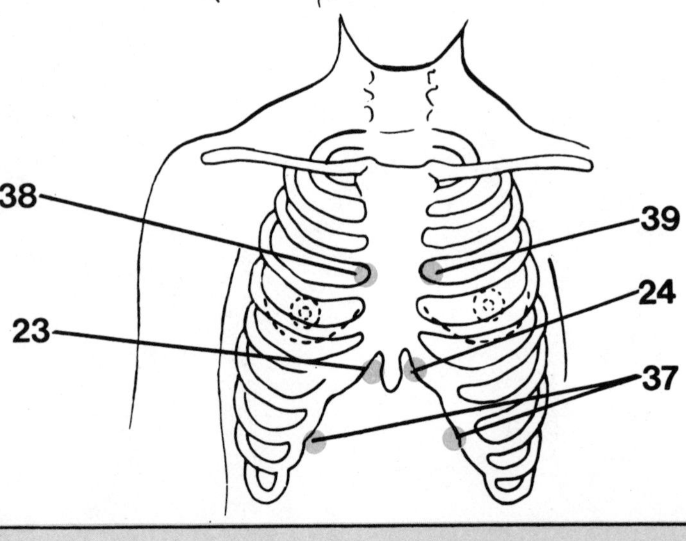

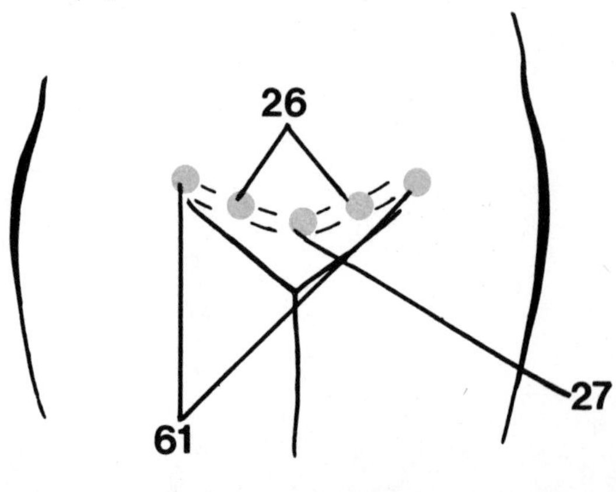

Points of the Body

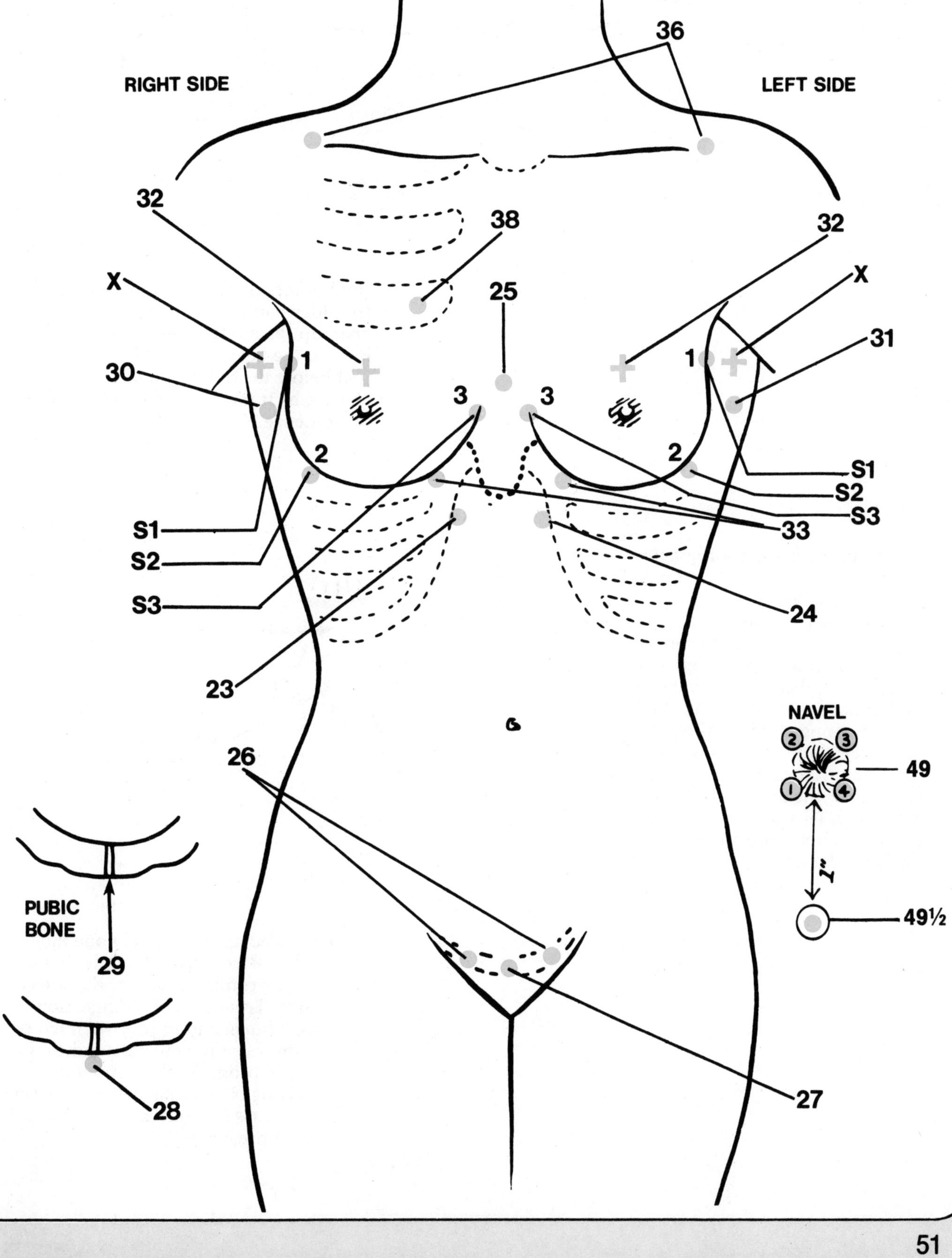

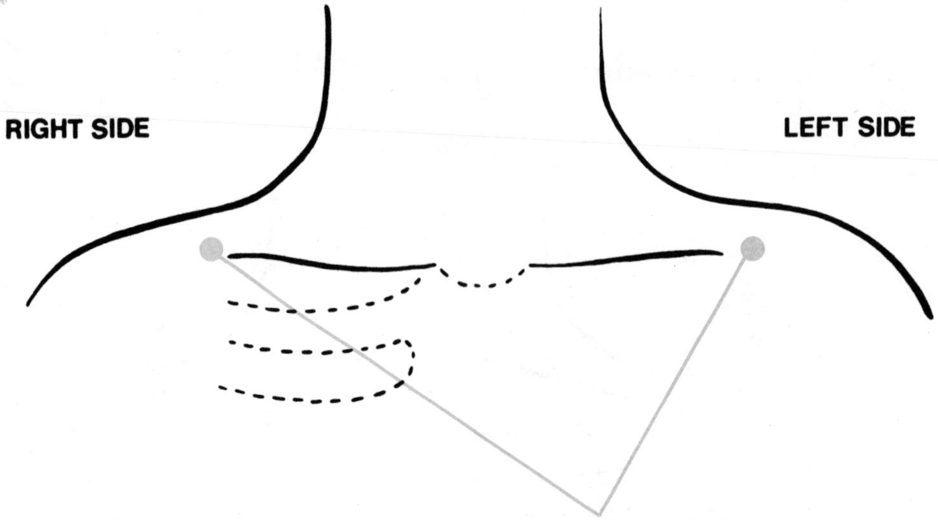

36 arm, neck and shoulder pains, breathing, circulation

Dual points treat arm, neck and shoulder pains, breathing, and open up the circulation from the liver to the heart. They are located just below the distal end of the clavicle as it meets the shoulder prominence.

7 bladder, dropsy, ribs, thymus

On the anterior superior quarter of the breastbone, or sternum, will be found on palpation, a bony ridge, or protuberance, that goes across it from one side to the other. Just above the center of this landmark is the contact that goes to that portion of the small intestines affecting abdominal bloat, water retention and dropsy, a condition that causes excessive swelling of the ankles and legs with fluid. This contact also goes to the thymus gland and treats the ribs and bladder.

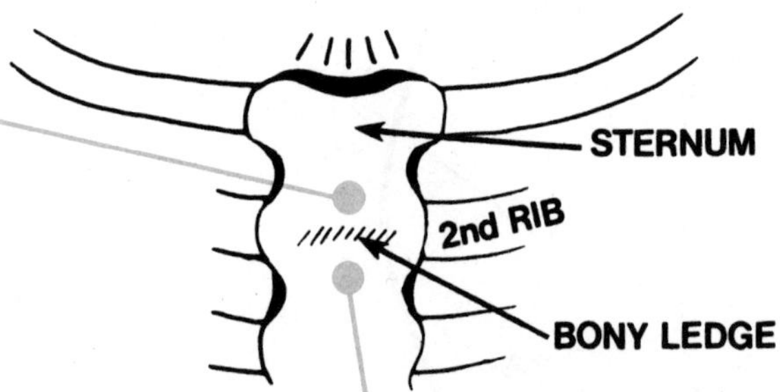

8 acid indigestion, breathing, heart pressure, mucous

Located approximately one inch below #7 or just below the bony ledge prominent across the breastbone. Treat for acid indigestion, heartburn, and to release mucous from the stomach and conditions or symptoms such as coughing, hiccoughs, asthma and diphtheria. Contact #8 also treats the ribs and heart pressure.

38 gallbladder, heart valves, pancreas

Located on the right side between the third and fourth ribs against join the sternum. This point treats the gallbladder, certain types of constipation, heart valves, the pancreas and the right phrenic and vagus nerves.

39 heart valves, mucous

A single contact, located between the third and fourth ribs against the left side of the sternum or breastbone. This contact is used to treat mucous in bronchi, intestines and colon, the left vagus and phrenic nerves and the heart valves.

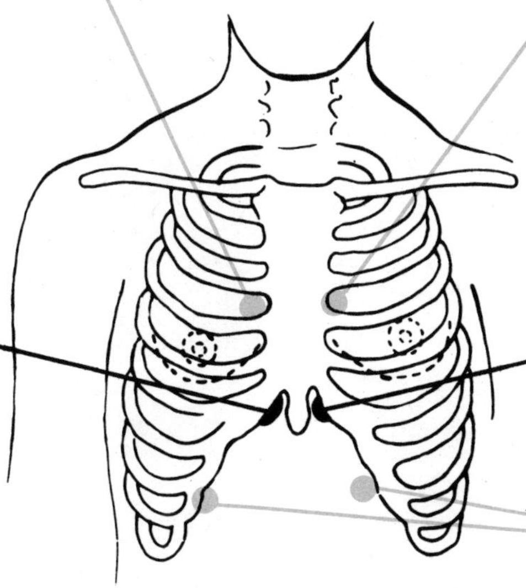

37 ANTERIOR RIB CAGE
fast heart, urine retention

Dual points at the bottom of the ribs which contact kidneys, ureters and bladder and are located by hooking the finger along the inside margin of the ribs approximately two-thirds of the distance down from the lowest end of the breastbone or sternum.

Generally, a slight notch in the rib margin will indicate that you have the correct contact. Treat for all types of urine retention. Dropsy, ascites, anasarca, gas and even indigestion can originate in kidney malfunction. These points also help a fast heart.

Prolapsed or fallen abdominal organs can also cause dropsy and hernia. Always check the 15B first (see page 46) to see if the abdominal organs need lifting to remove pressure. 33's are for kidney pain (see page 56).

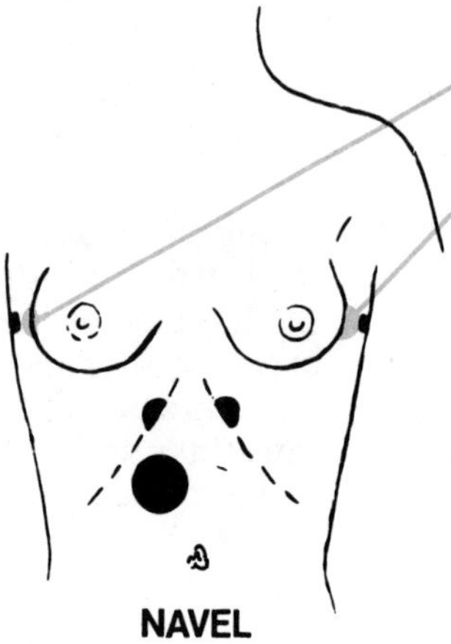

56 reproductive system

#30 and #31 are under each arm, level with the nipples of the breasts. The 56's are just in front of those two numbers, right in the edge of the breasts. These 56's are master contacts to the entire reproductive system of both man and woman: the breasts, ovaries, prostate, spermatic cords, testes, tubes, uterus, thyroid and the neck. The reproductive organs can affect the emotional system.

95 heart

Use this contact for the heart. It is located between the 5th and 6th ribs below each breast, and affects the hormones to the heart.

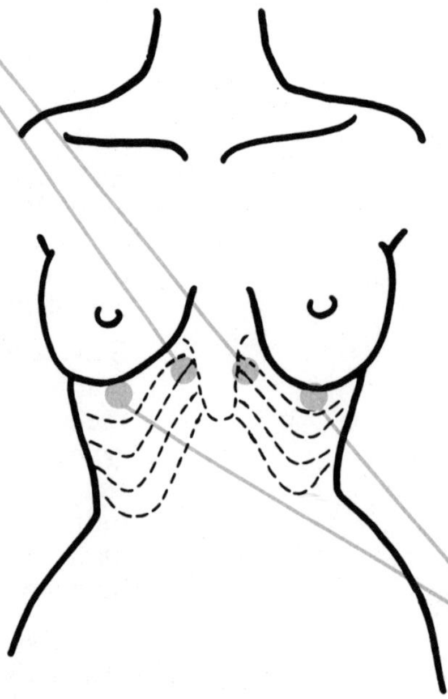

96 bronchi, lungs

These contacts treat the greater part of the lungs and bronchi. They are located directly below each nipple under each breast.

66 back pain, lungs

Located between the clavicle and the first rib adjacent to the sternum. Treat for lungs and bronchi (the upper part of the lungs); also for back pain.

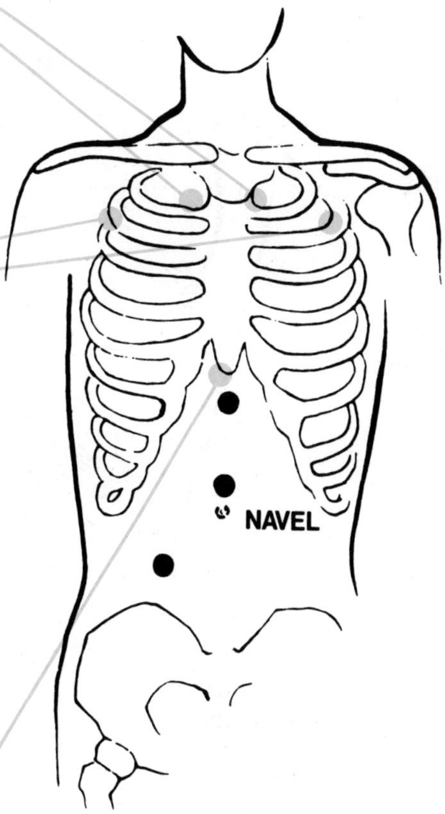

ANTERIOR ASPECT

64 ***Systemic***
arterial circulation, tetanus, tobacco poisoning

Located on each side of the upper thoracic region on the end of each second rib where it passes under the collarbone. It influences arterial circulation in lungs, intestines and colon. It is especially indicated in tobacco poisoning and tetanus.

67 venous congestion

Located on the tip of the breastbone. For venous congestion.

X *right*
venous blood

X *left*
arterial blood

For venous and arterial blood. The left "X" is located in the axilla of the left arm at the highest point one can comfortably touch against these ribs. This contacts all the arterial blood through the aorta, heart and body. The contact on the right "X" is the same as under the left arm, only this one contacts all the venous blood through the portal circulation and liver. Use both for lymphatic congestion also.

25 heart

Located in the center of the sternum or breastbone directly between the nipples of each breast. It affects the right side of the heart. (A single contact.)

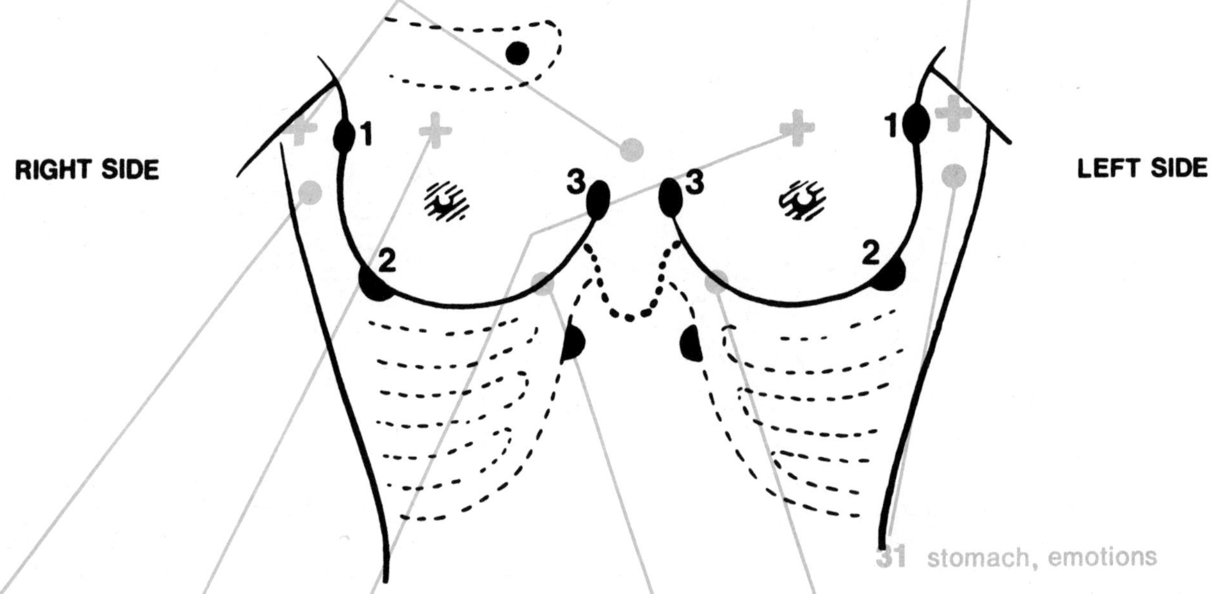

30 liver

Level with the right nipple, but under the right arm, against the rib, this is one of three contacts to the liver.

31 stomach, emotions

For the stomach. It is located on a level with the left nipple, on the left rib cage, under the arm.

33 *left*
left kidney and colon

32 *left*
arteries to colon, intestines, heart

33 *right*
right kidney and colon

On the right side this contact treats the right kidney and the right side of the colon. On the left side it treats the left kidney and the left side of the colon. Located under and against the under side of each breast on the ribs at a point midway between the lowest part of the breast and the point where the breast touches the breastbone or sternum. For kidney pains.

32 *right*
veins to colon and intestines

On the right side, #32 treats the veins to the colon and intestines, and is located approximately two inches directly superior to the right nipple. Left 32 above the left nipple treats the arteries to the colon, intestines and heart.

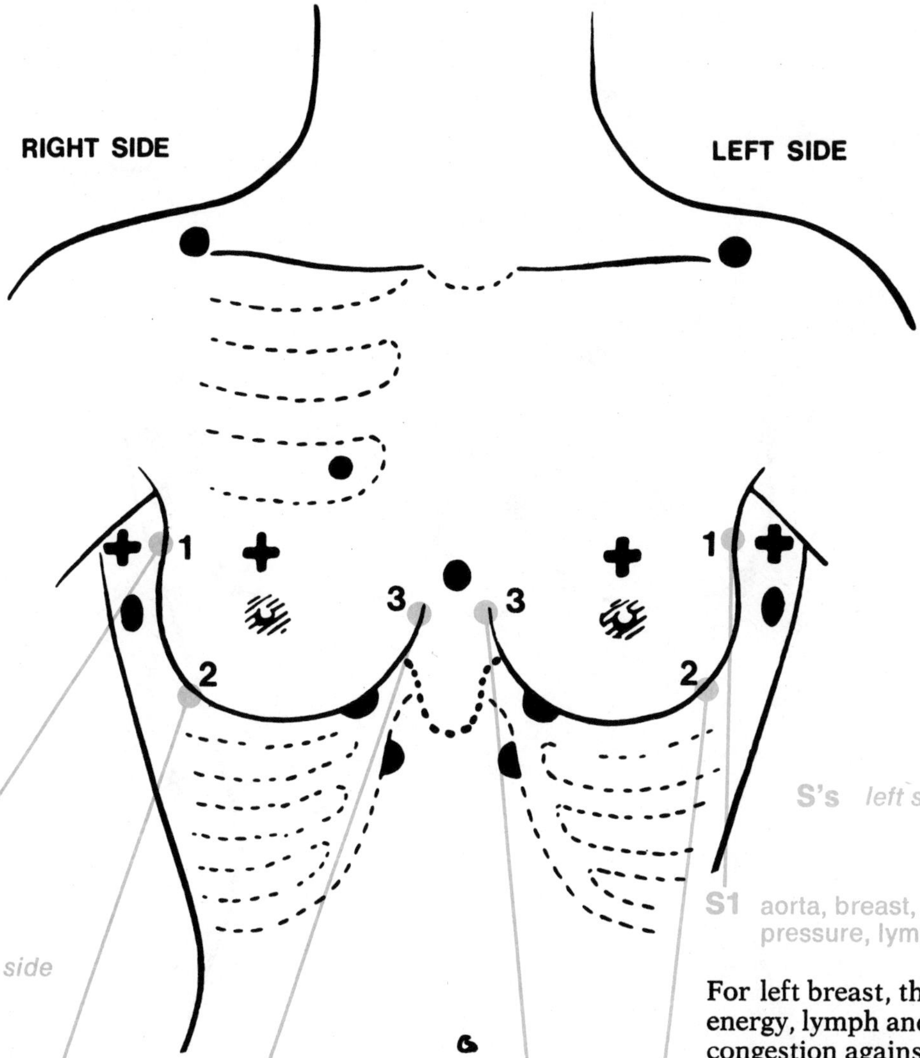

S's *right side*

S1 acid indigestion, breast, veins

For right breast and all the veins. This is one to remember with the 12M's (see page 33) in case of shock. It is also to be used for acid indigestion. Contact by pressing with fingertip directly in the center of the breast muscles as they leave the anterior aspect of each arm.

S2 breast, liver

For breast and liver. Located under the lateral side of the breast against the rib.

S3 breast, ears, deafness, tinnitus, liver

For breast, liver and the ears, especially deafness and tinnitus. It is located right at the points where the breast muscle joins the breastbone or sternum.

S's *left side*

S1 aorta, breast, energy, heart pressure, lymph

For left breast, the aorta, energy, lymph and arterial congestion against the left side of the heart. Located the same as S1 on the right side.

S2 breast, heart congestion and pressure, lymph

For breast, lymph and relieves congestion and pressure from beneath the heart. Located the same as S2 on the right side.

S3 breast, bloat, ears, heart pressure, indigestion, lymph, stomach, rectum

For breast, lymph and relieves pressure against the right side of the heart. S3 also for ear troubles such as deafness and tinnitus; abdominal bloat; dropsy; water retention; excess fluid; pain in the rectum and anus and many digestive problems—acid indigestion, heartburn, belching, gas, dyspepsia and nausea. It is located the same as S3 on the right side.

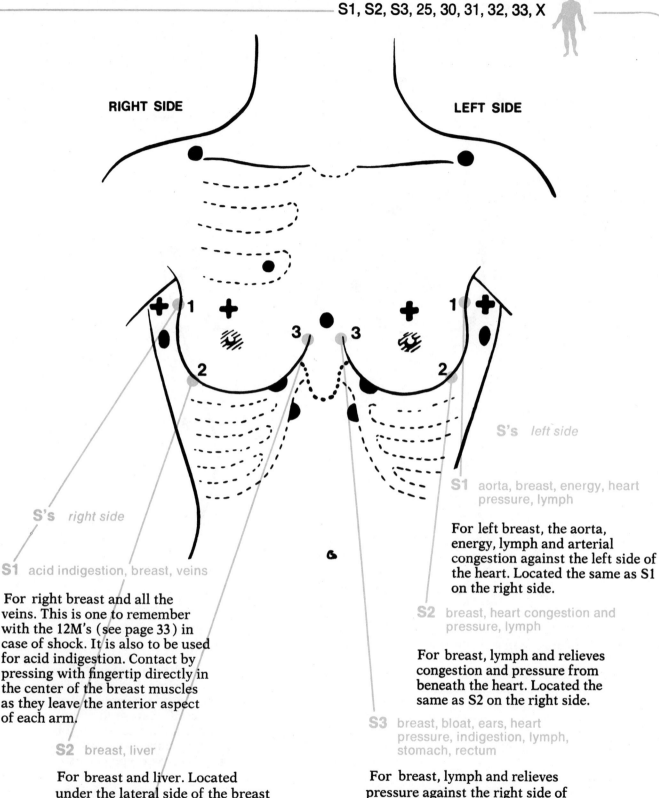

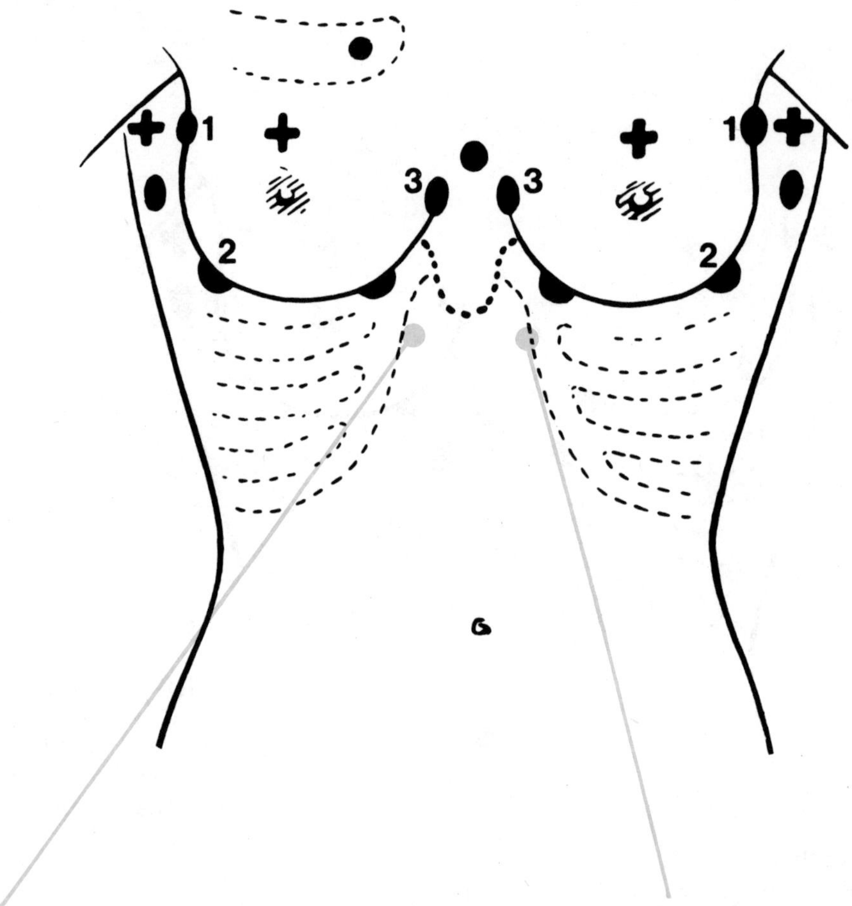

23 pancreas

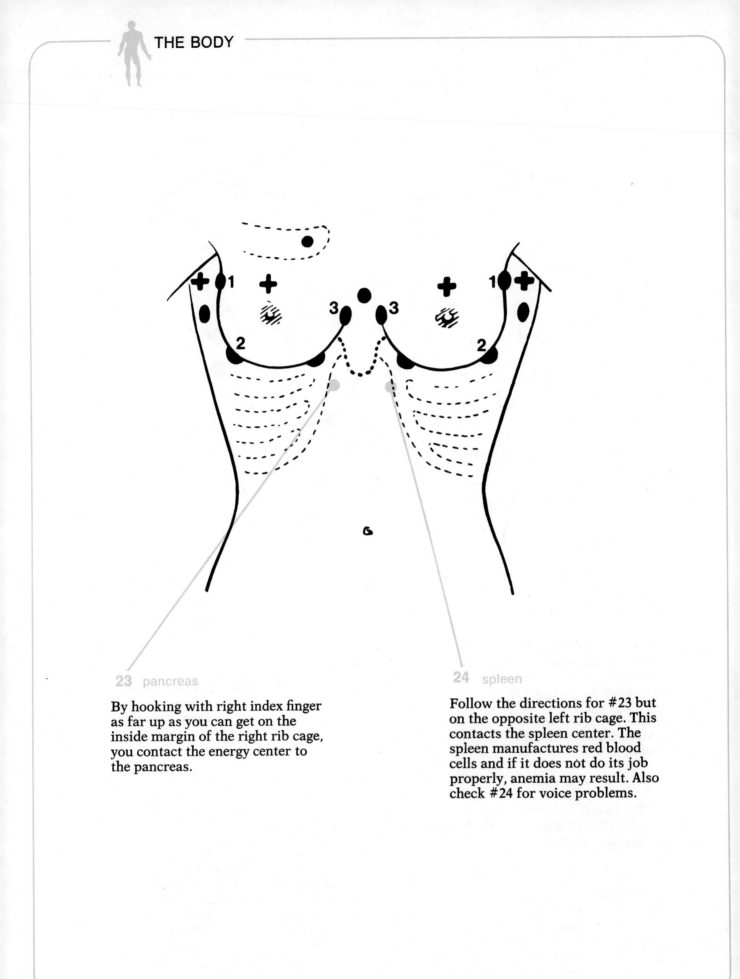

By hooking with right index finger as far up as you can get on the inside margin of the right rib cage, you contact the energy center to the pancreas.

24 spleen

Follow the directions for #23 but on the opposite left rib cage. This contacts the spleen center. The spleen manufactures red blood cells and if it does not do its job properly, anemia may result. Also check #24 for voice problems.

54 bile, digestion, gallstones

On the right side, approximately two to three inches directly below the Right #37 on the abdominal wall, press straight down against the tissue. This is not something felt on the outside tissues but deep within. Use some care, however, as in some cases great tenderness may indicate that there is congestion in the bile duct, the tube leading from the gall bladder to the intestines. Since bile is most essential for all fat digestion, you can see how important it is to keep this passageway opened. A small stone can obstruct this passage to the intestine.

88 constipation, fast heart

Located exactly the same as #54 but on the opposite side of the abdomen. This is the contact that releases the contents of the intestines. Treat for constipation. If #54 is painful also, then treat both together. Number 88 is also a specific contact for a fast heart.

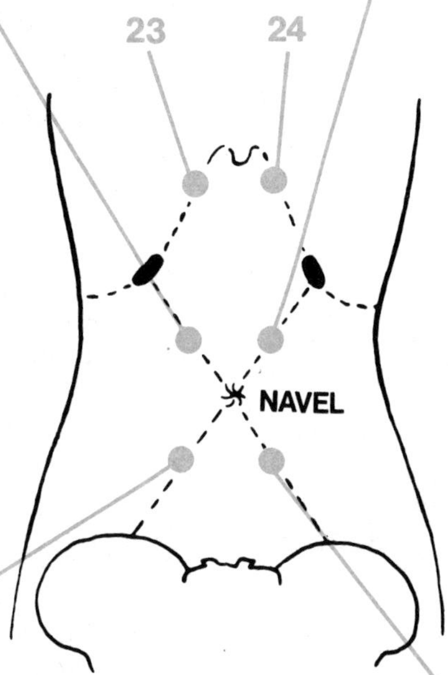

65 appendicitis, colon, insulin

Located midway between the crest of the right hip bone and the navel. This point has always been called "McBurnie's" point and is a medical diagnostic point to determine appendicitis in a patient. It also seems to stimulate colon gas and increase mobility of the colon and strongly influences distribution of insulin.

93 constipation

Located in the same position as the appendix contact #65, but on the opposite side of the lower abdomen. This #93 contacts the sigmoid flexure or outlet of the colon just before the rectum or anus. For constipation due to congestion in this area of the colon.

UMBILICUS OR NAVEL

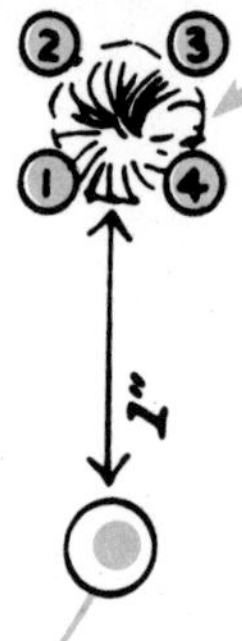

49 abdominal aorta, digestion, heart, mental problems

Through the umbilicus, or navel, the life fluids are carried to the unborn child until its birth. After birth this navel area remains of vital importance to the continuing life of the entity because directly around it, and touching it, are four contacts that keep the duodenum or first twelve inches of the small intestine in working order.

The duodenum, as it leaves the lower or pyloric valve of the stomach, is the seat or very heart of our digestive process. It is here that the arterial blood picks up the electrical force of our food and drink and carries it to every part of our body and brain. Therefore, as you need treatment for these #49 contacts you may also feel the influence of the treatment referring to any other part, or parts, of the body or brain. Consider #49 in all digestive problems, gas and indigestion, duodenal ulcers, the utilization of calcium, and oil, fat, sugar and starch digestion, heart cases, chronic back pains and mental problems. Even a baby can have trouble at these points because of very poor nutritional habits of the mother during pregnancy.

Remember this—the best food in the world can and will destroy you if you can't digest it. . . . There are four contacts which make up #49. Each contact treats approximately three inches of the duodenum and are numbered 1, 2, 3 and 4. The #3 and #4 on the left side of the navel also treat the abdominal aorta and you will feel the strong pulse of it under your finger as you treat.

Check also the gall bladder and bile ducts—#38 (see page 53) and #54, (see page 59) also the pancreas—#14B (see page 41) and #23 (see page 58).

49½ abdominal swelling, bone-marrow of hipbones, lungs

Directly inferior to, or below, the navel at a distance of approximately one inch, will be found another center or contact that is most powerful in maintaining life forces by its action on the bone marrow of the large hip bones which in turn radiates energy up through both lungs. Also check this contact in all abdominal swellings. Many people have chronic hip pains that are in reality only referral pains from an imbalance of life forces in the marrow of the bone, or a lung problem on the same side. Congestion of the left lung can result in one form of heart imbalance and dizziness.

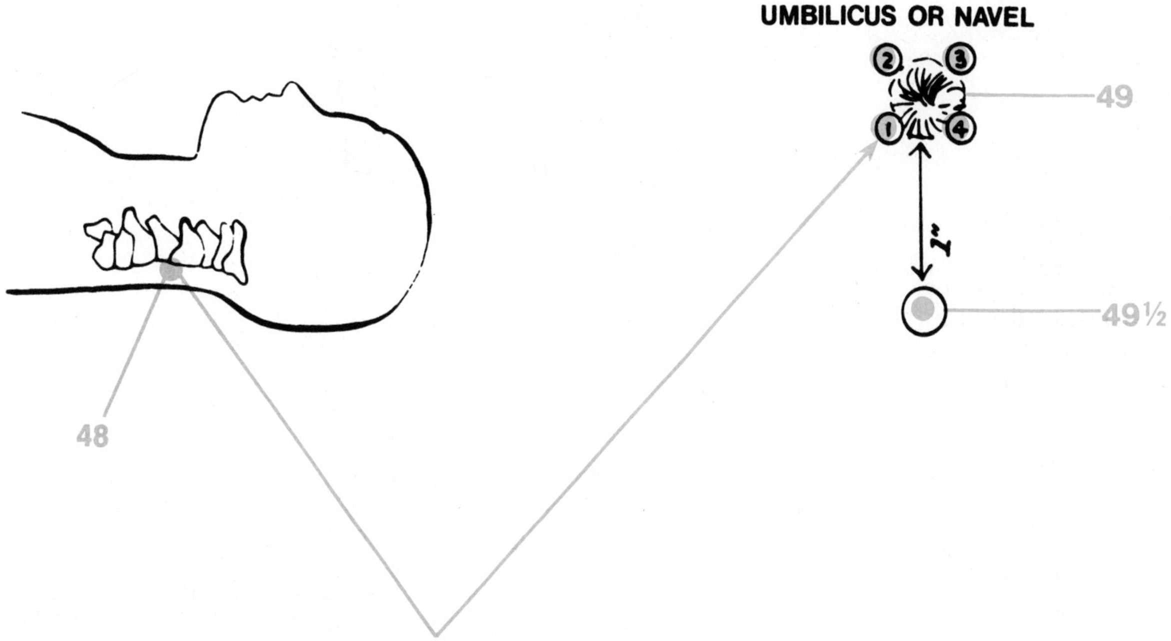

60 constipation

This is a combination of two contacts (#48 and the navel) made simultaneously with both hands.

Contact #48 with the index finger of one hand, then place the thumb of the other hand in the navel (umbilicus) of the body and hold both simultaneously with a firm contact. Great warmth should build up in the lower abdomen.

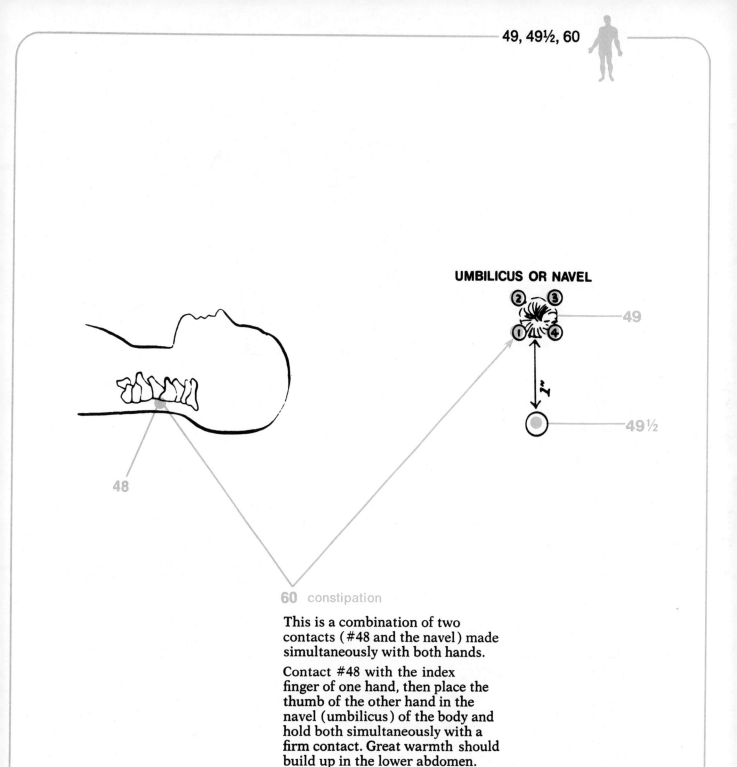

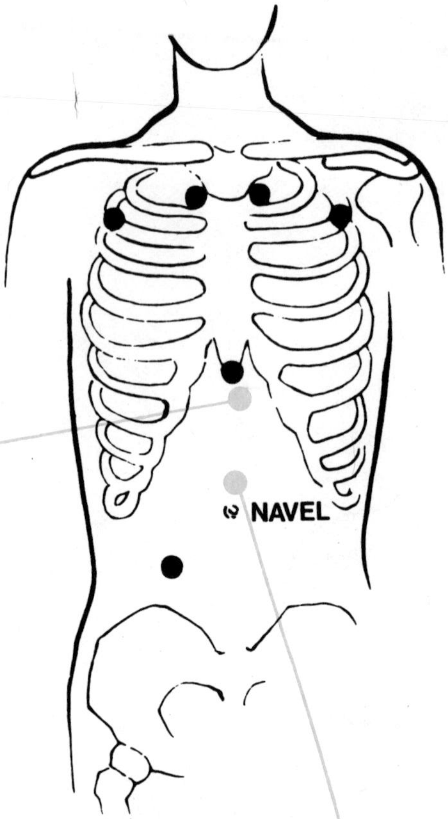

ANTERIOR ASPECT

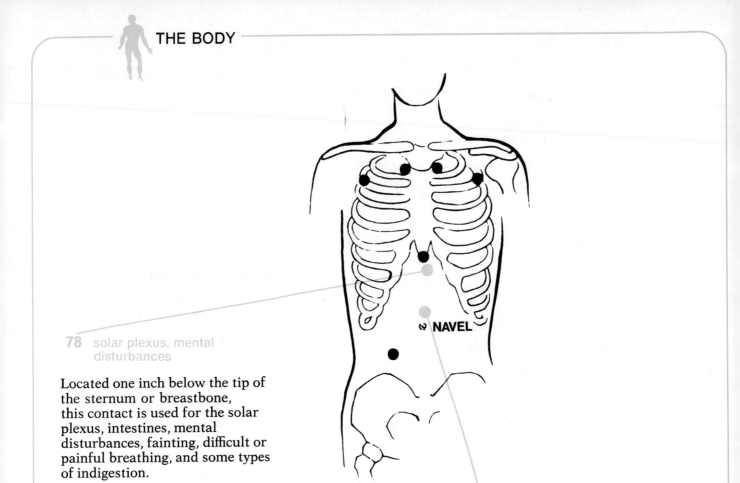

78 solar plexus, mental disturbances

Located one inch below the tip of the sternum or breastbone, this contact is used for the solar plexus, intestines, mental disturbances, fainting, difficult or painful breathing, and some types of indigestion.

62 bladder, energy, worry

Located two inches above the navel. Influences the solar plexus and is specific for incontinence of urine as well as urine retention, bedwetting, worry, body energy and shock.

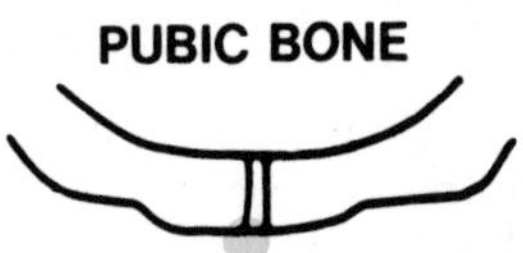

28 water retention

With the index finger under and adjacent to #27, press straight in a posterior direction. This treats the ureter and bladder.

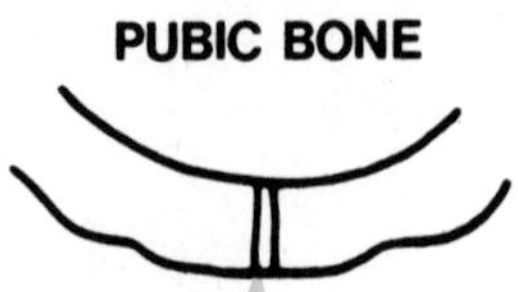

29 penis or vagina

With the index finger just under and adjacent to #27, press upward against the under side of contact #27. This is the contact point to the vagina or penis.

61 circulation

Located in each groin on the beginning of the pubic bones. Tenderness or pain on these contacts indicates lack of circulation from the legs and feet to the heart. In varicose veins, leg ulcers, and other leg and feet conditions, #61 contacts should be checked first.

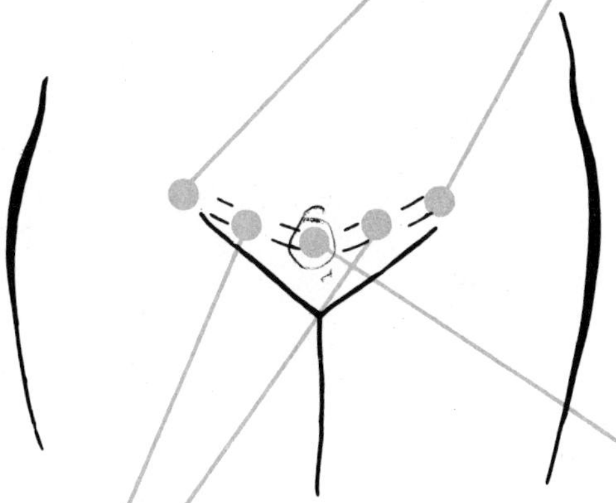

27 prostate or uterus

A single contact, located exactly in the middle, where the two pubic bones come together. This contact treats the uterus in the female, the prostate in the male and the neck.

26 ovaries, tubes, spermatic cords

This contact is dual, being located in the center of each pubic bone, and it treats the ovaries and tubes in the female, the spermatic cords in the male and the neck. One of the main symptoms of congestion in the reproductive organs is pain in the legs and low back and even, in some cases, the inability to walk. If congestion in these organs cannot be released by treatment on the contact centers, check contact #51 (see page 39) as mumps may have left their mark in the testes or ovaries. The reproductive organs are composed of sensitive nerves, hence the emotional symptoms arising from troubles in these areas, such as the nervous difficulties during menopause.

The Back
and its Pressure Points

The 15 Pressure

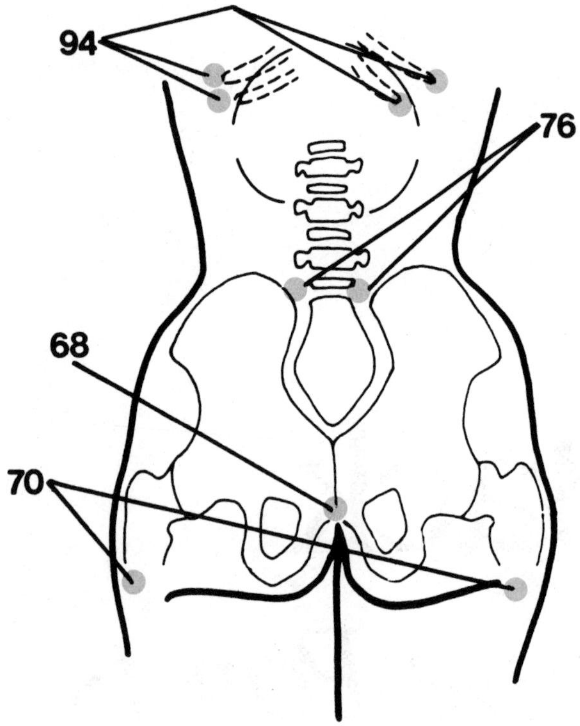

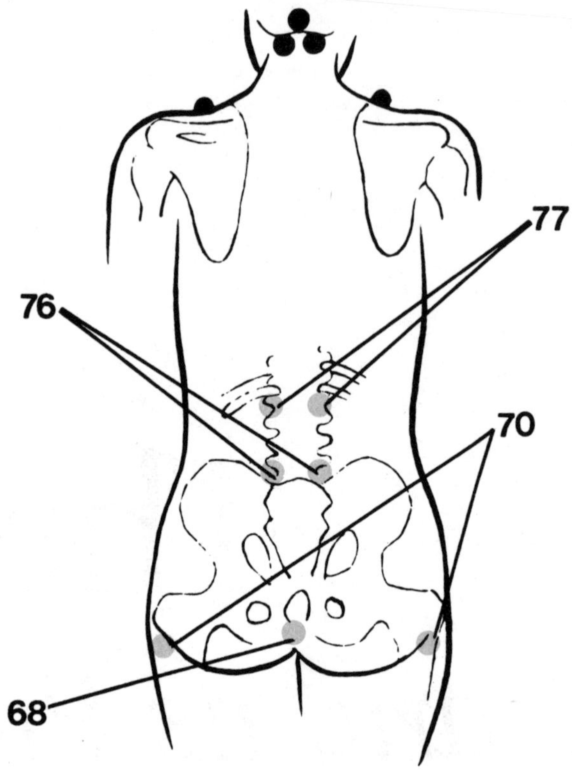

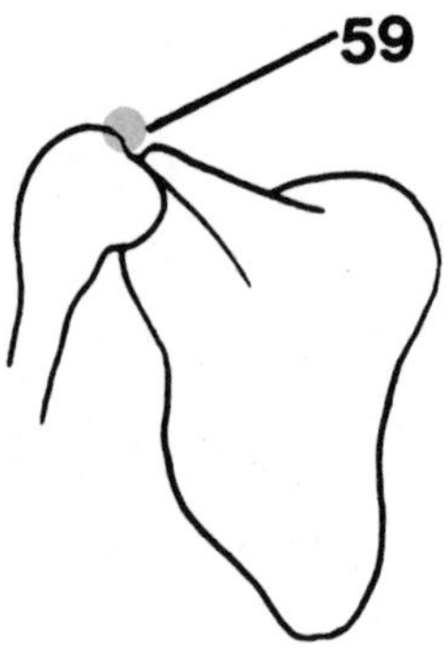

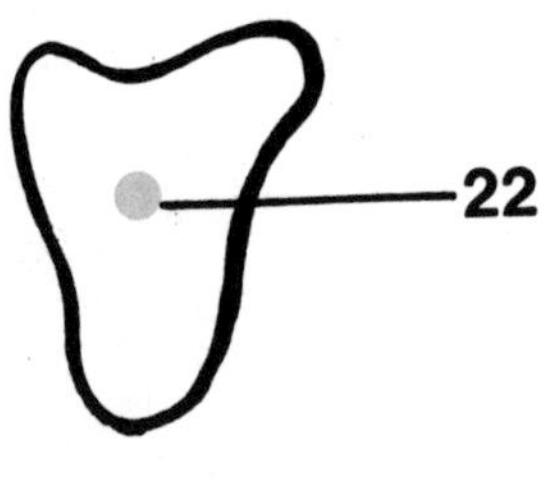

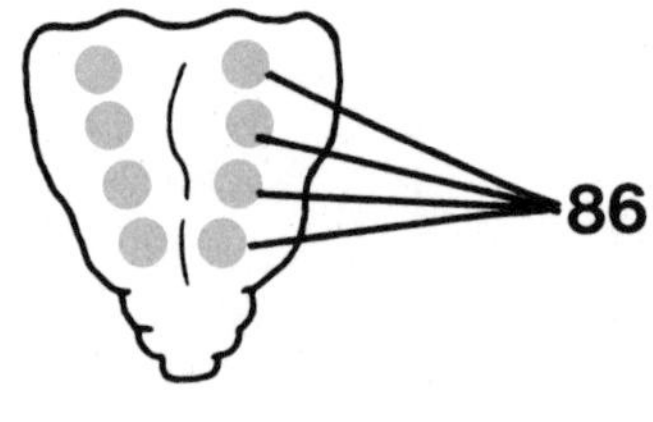

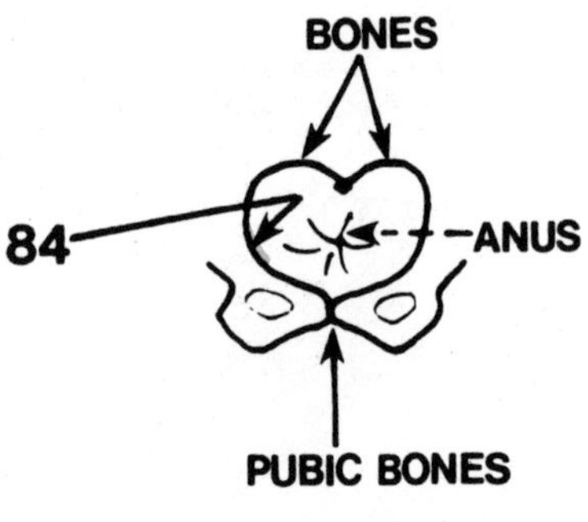

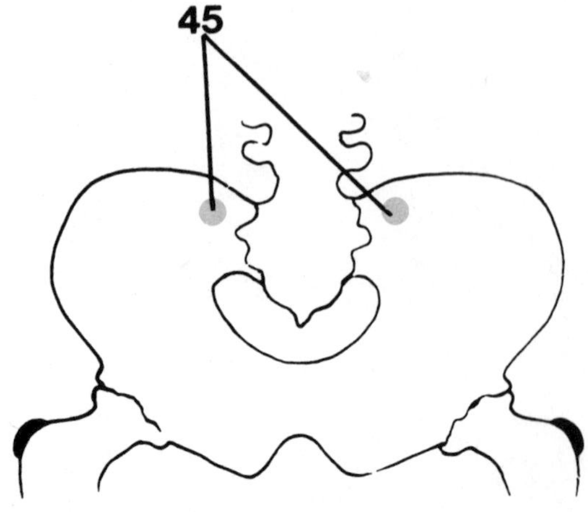

Points of the Back

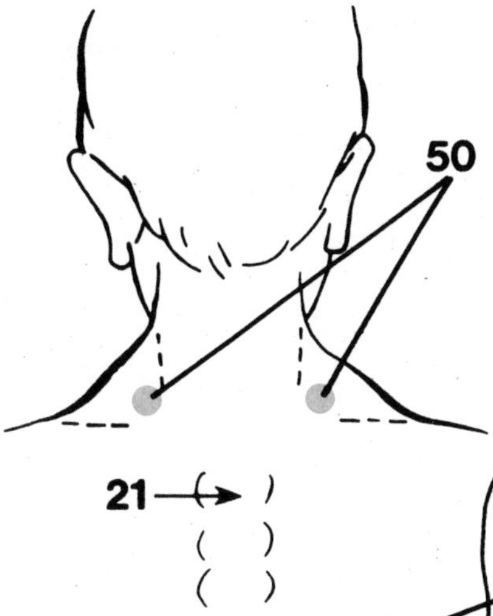

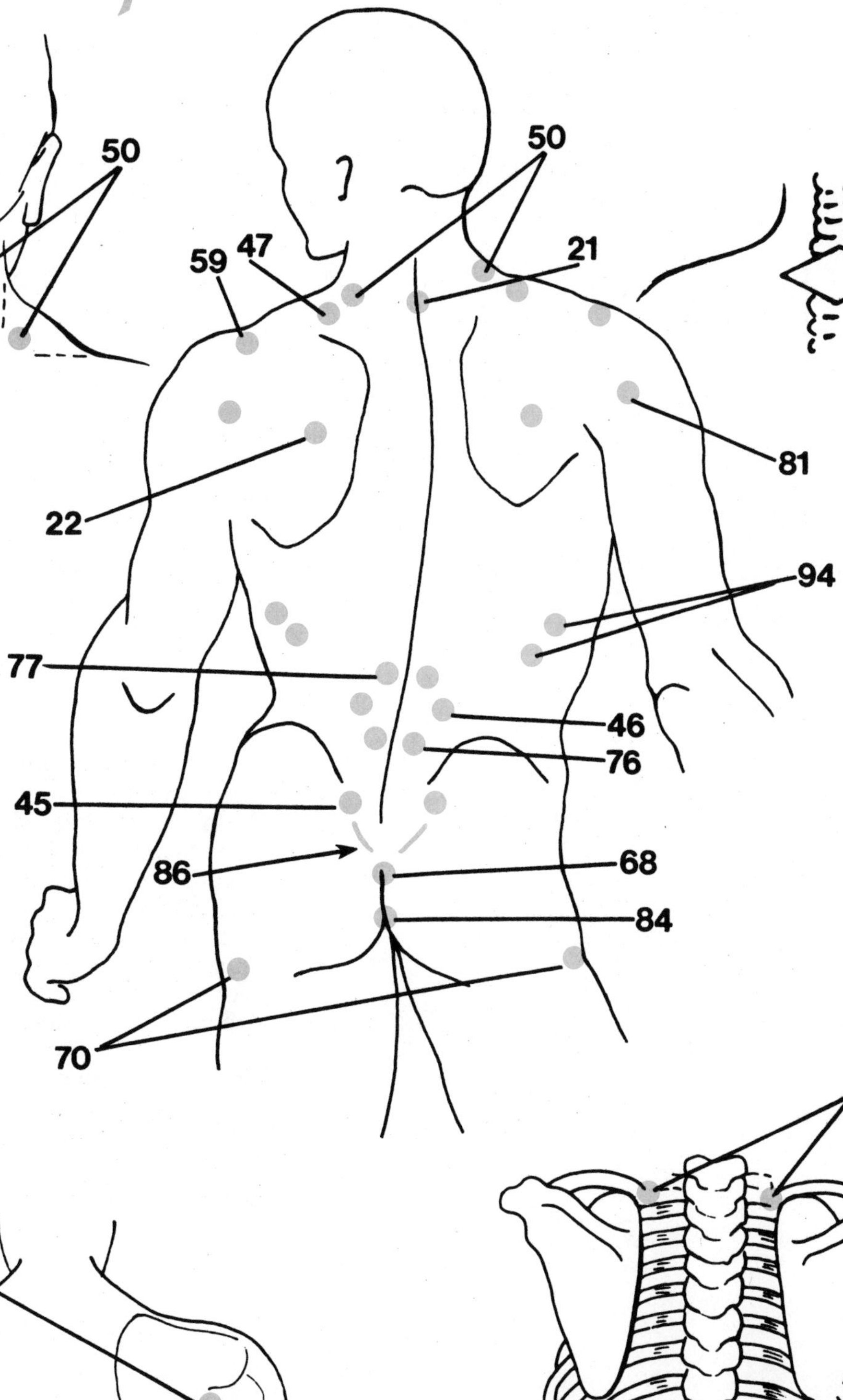

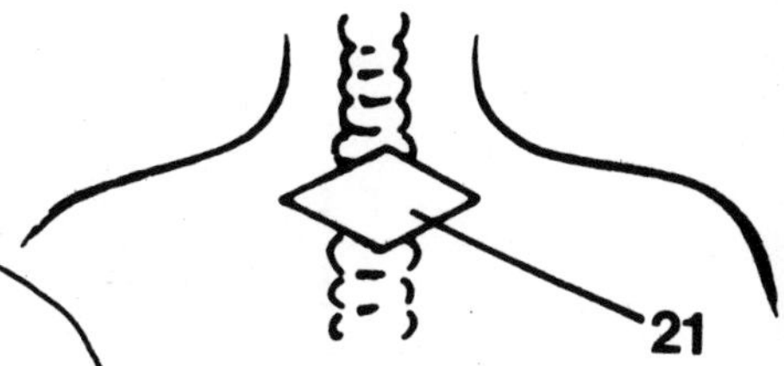

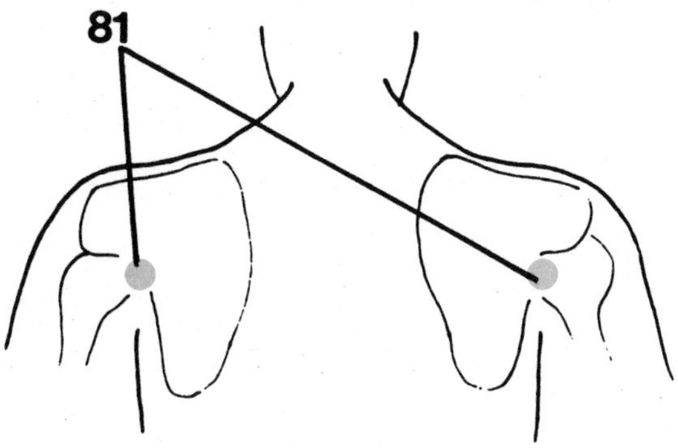

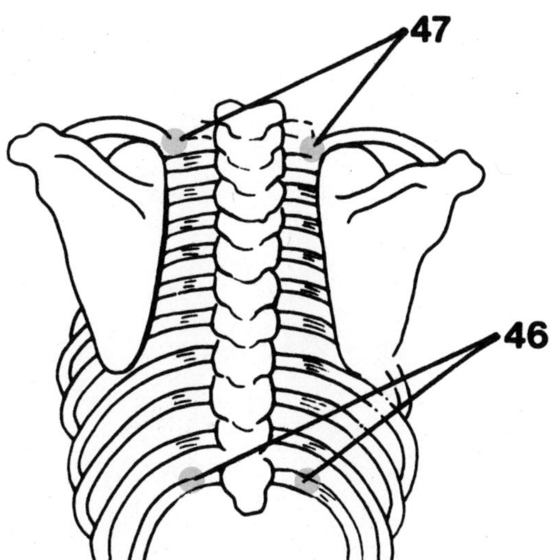

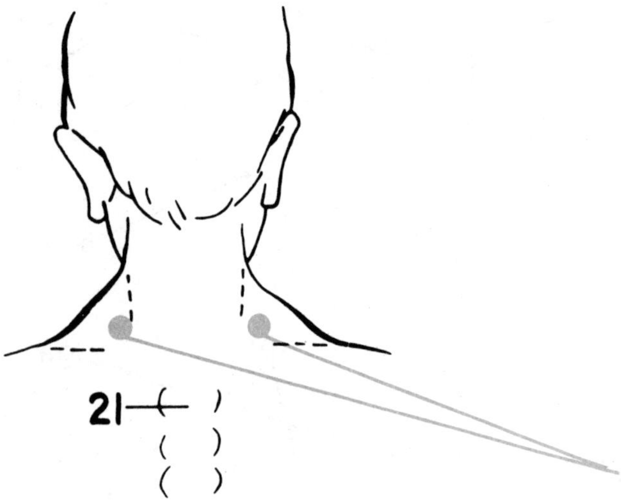

50 *Systemic*
diabetes, tension

Ask a friend or family member to stand behind you and place his thumbs at the base of your neck on each side simultaneously. Press inward and down at approximately a 45-degree angle, directing the contact toward #21. This contact is painful in everyone because everyone today suffers from tension. To release congestion in neck and brain and for mental fatigue. Also used to sober up an alcoholic (JB10's are also used for this purpose [see page 39]) and for insomnia and diabetes.

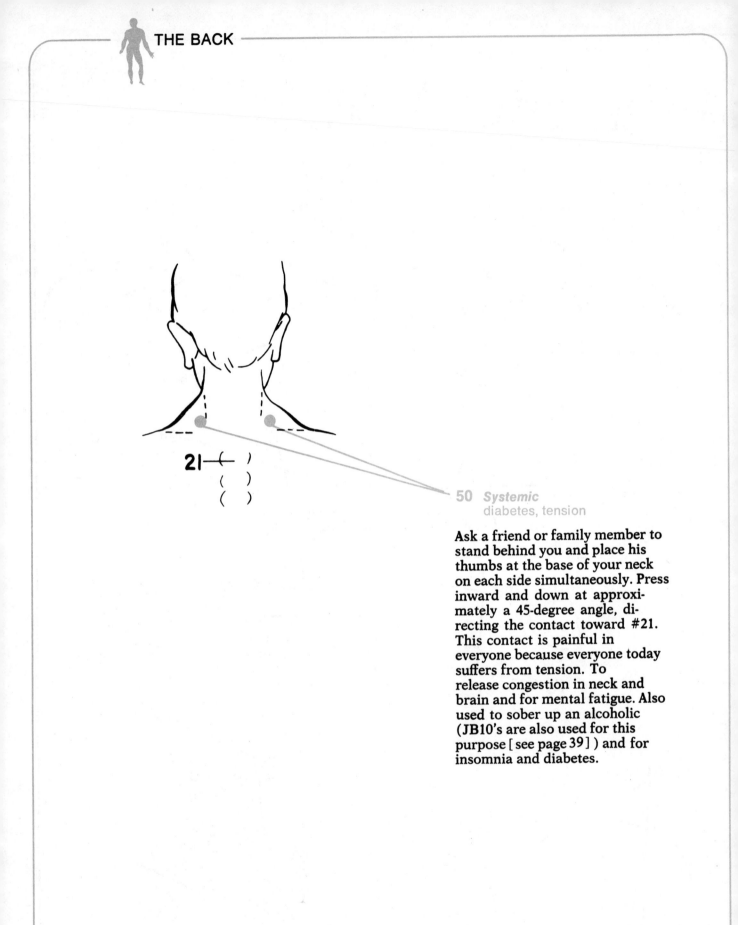

47 spastic or painful arms, legs, hips

These contacts are located on the superior aspect of each scapula or shoulder blade. Check contact at approximate area where second rib passes under the scapula. Helps to release hip and leg pains —also spastic conditions of legs and arms.

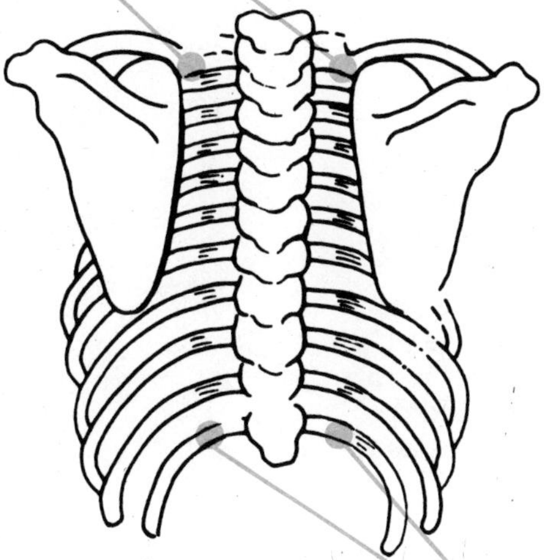

46 heart, breathing, pain

Located on the bottom of the rib cage (or 12th rib) approximately three inches on either side of the spine. I cannot overstress the value of these contacts as adrenalin is of vital importance to the life of every cell in our body. For heart cases, difficult breathing and pain in any part of the body, especially hip and leg pains.

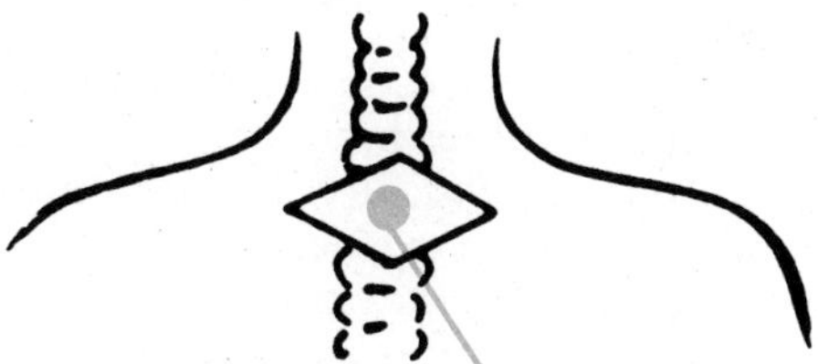

21 7th CERVICLE VERTEBRA
bones, heart, spine

Situated on the spinous process of the 7th cervical vertebra where the neck joins the shoulders. This is the body contact to the pituitary, thyroid and every bone in the body. If you fracture or break a bone, contact #21 becomes very painful. 21 is for relief. Also for heart, spinal cord and spinal nerves.

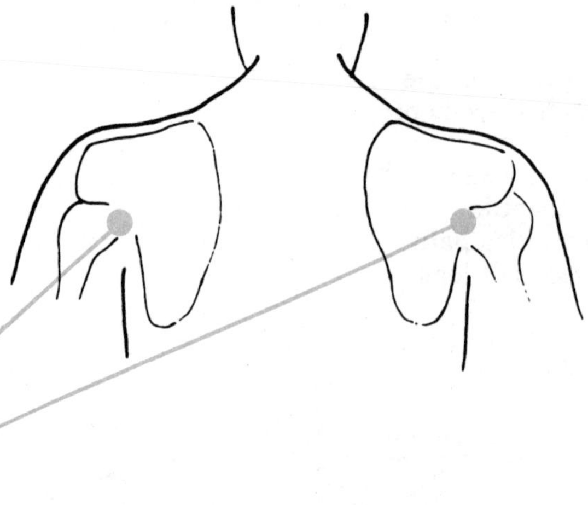

81 bursitis

Located in the posterior part of the shoulder joint. Study diagram closely. It is a contact that is practically impossible to do on one's self, but is perhaps one of the most important contact points for bursitis and other shoulder and arm pains. Also, if necessary, treat Left #15M (see page 47) or #40 (see page 86).

59 apoplexy, injuries, fatigue, shock

The 59's may seem a little difficult to find at first. Have someone else stand behind you while you are seated. With his thumbs he should follow outward the upper margin of the shoulder blade, or scapula, to the very end. It will feel blunt, not sharp, on each end when he locates it. He may place his thumb on each 59 and press inward toward the spine.

Consider these contacts in all cases of apoplexy, bruised or crushed tissue anywhere on the body, all head injuries, no matter how old they are, physical fatigue and all types of shock, particularly electric shock and its after effect on the heart. (Have both contacts treated at the same time.)

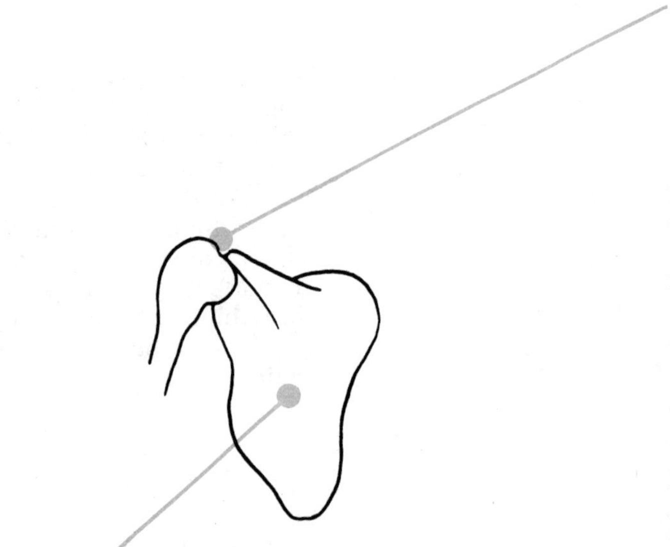

22 heart, lungs, flu

Dual contacts located in the center of each scapula or shoulder blade. They treat lungs, heart and some shoulder pains.

45 abdominal lymph

Located on each side of the crest of the sacrum on the ilium or hip bone. These contacts go to the insertion of the Achilles tendon, which in turn influences all the abdominal lymph. The lymph is a clear, colorless saline solution that bathes every cell in the body. It has no motive force like the heart to keep it moving. Its movement is controlled by action or physical movement of the body. The main activator of the abdominal lymph fluid is the Achilles tendon which runs from the back of the heel to muscles forming the calf of the leg, and thence up to the sacrum. Only one contact is more forceful in treating abdominal lymph: contact #73 (see page 82).

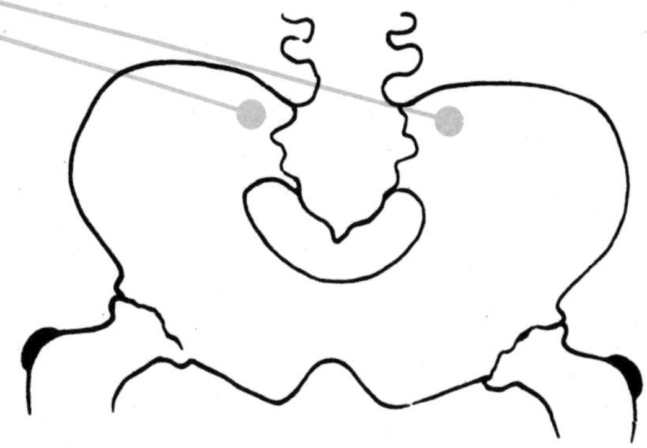

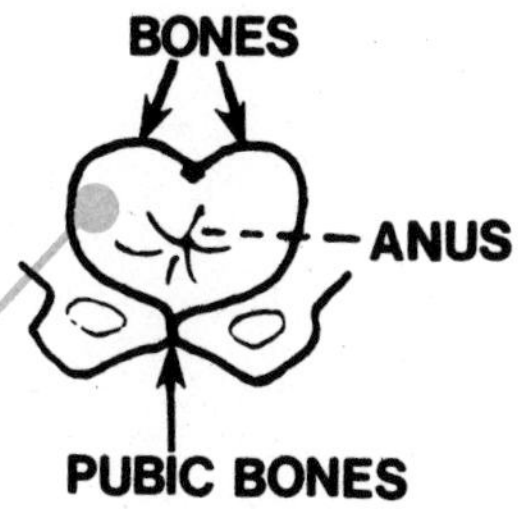

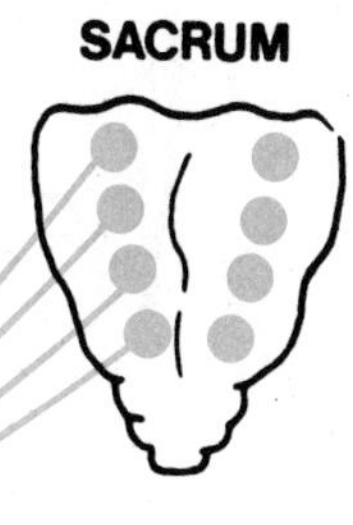

84 rectal pain

The inside margin of the lower pelvis makes a circle around the rectum and anus. Hook with your finger around the inside of this bony circle and in case of rectal pain, find a contact on this bone which responds. This circular bone is approximately two inches from anus on all sides. (Other contacts for rectal pain are #68 [see page 73] and #86).

86 SACRUM
sympathetic nervous system of back

The eight foramina or openings in the body of the sacrum. These are openings for nerves which are part of the sympathetic nervous system influencing the body from the rectum to the brain. Contact any of these which are painful. *Note*: Always check reproductive organs if sacral nerves are painful.

94

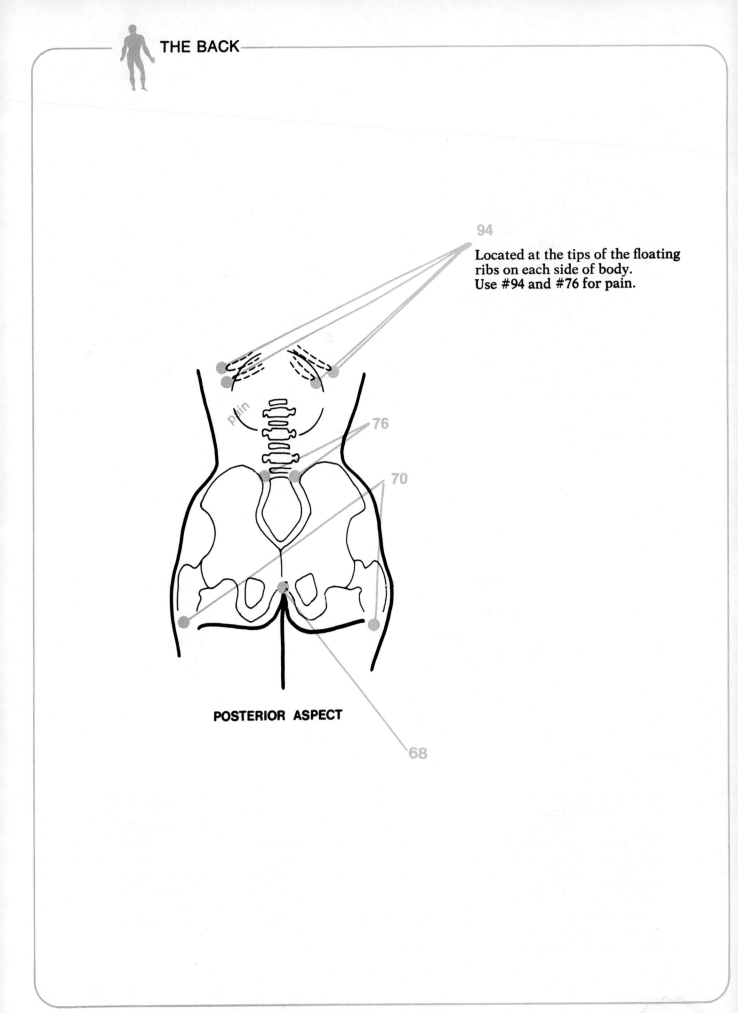

Located at the tips of the floating ribs on each side of body.
Use #94 and #76 for pain.

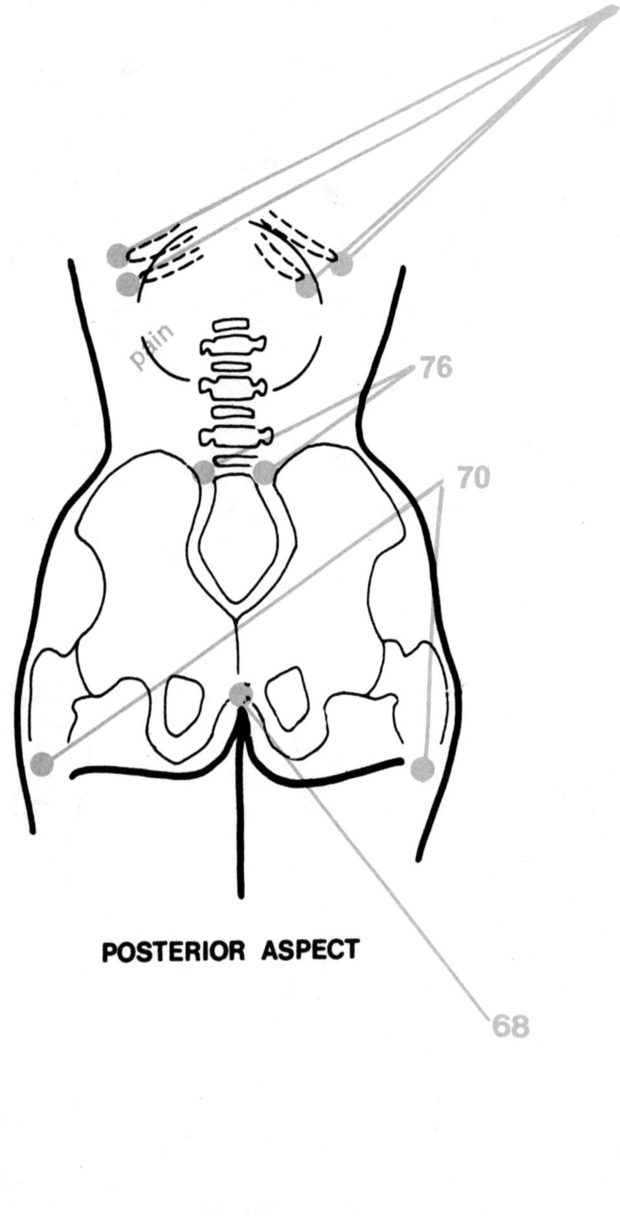

POSTERIOR ASPECT

77 *left*
abdomen, colon, stomach, thighs

77 *right*
appendix, gallbladder

Located on the transverse process of the 1st lumbar vertebra. Pressure on the right transverse releases congestion and pain in the gallbladder and appendix. Pressure on the left transverse releases tension in thighs, abdomen, colon and stomach.

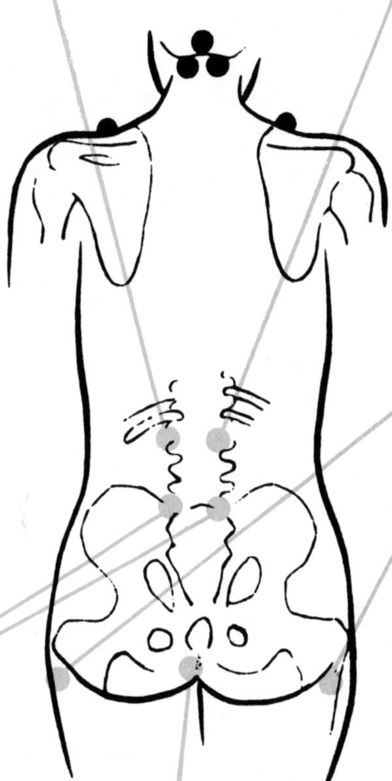

70 colon, leg pains

Lie face down. Have someone else follow the curve of the buttocks downward until the posterior upper thigh is contacted. Then with the tip of the thumbs, press through the upper leg tissue to the posterior surface of the femur bone. Check for pain on one or both of these contacts for colon trouble and leg pains.

POSTERIOR ASPECT

76 tension in abdomen and hip, leg pains

Located on the transverse processes of the 5th lumbar vertebra. Treat for tension in abdomen and hip and for leg pains. (Also treat contacts #94.)

68 coccyx
energy, stomach

Located on the tip of the coccyx bone. The coccyx bone reflects energy through pelvic and reproductive organs, stomach and brain. Press tip of coccyx toward head and hold. Also treat for stomach trouble.

The Arms and Legs

and their Pressure Points

The 25 Pressure
Arms

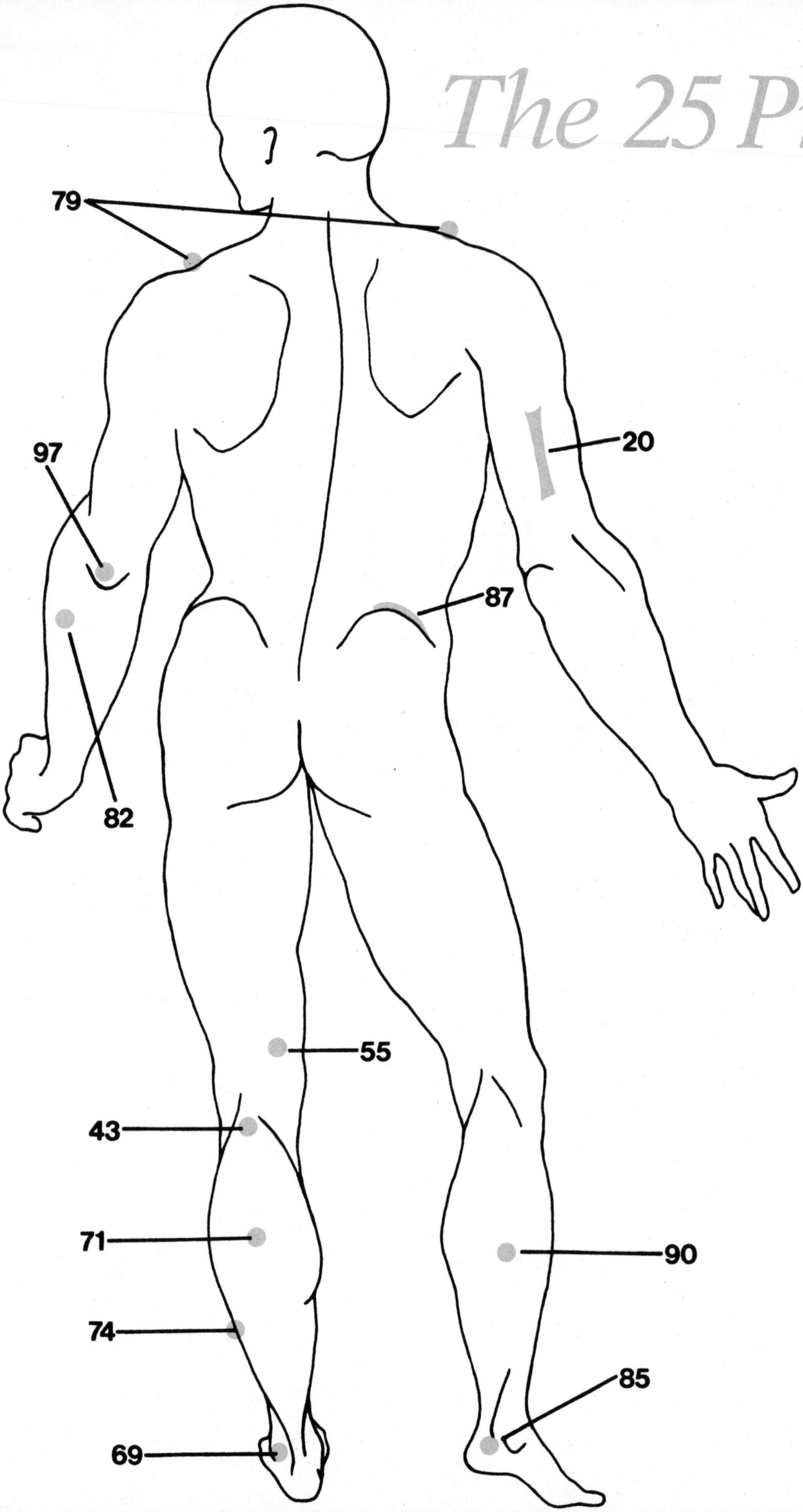

Points of the
and Legs

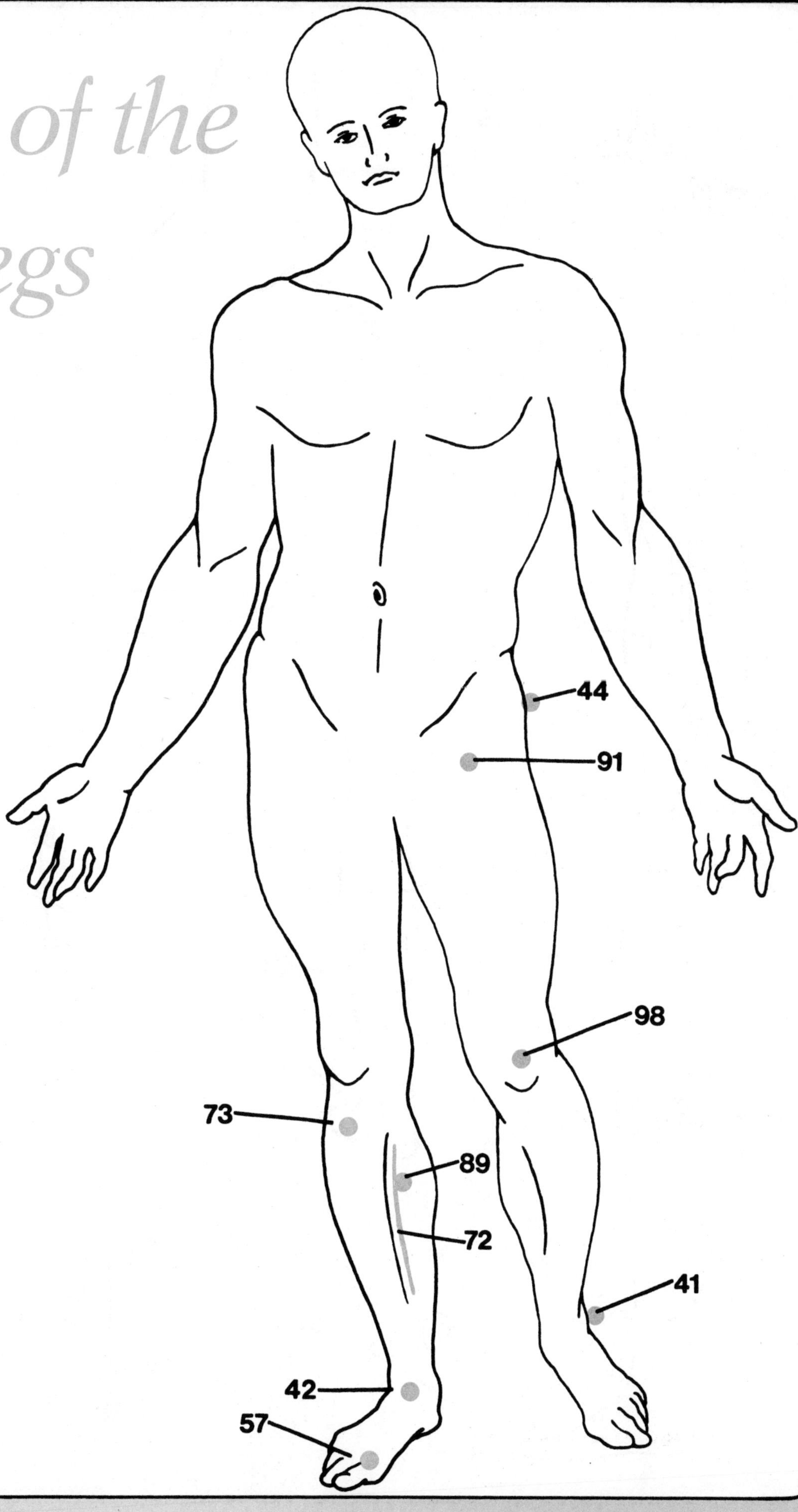

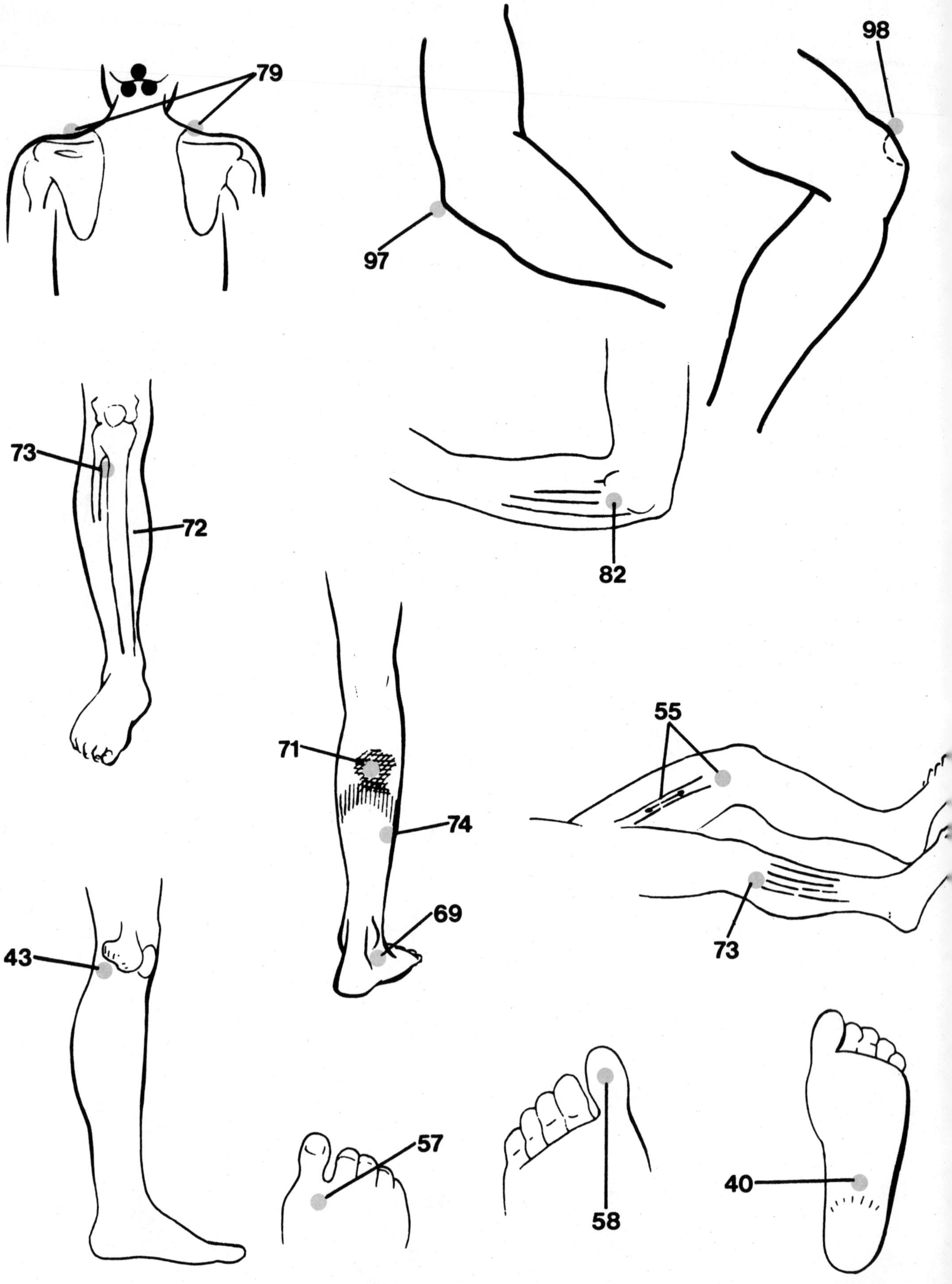
79
98
97
73
72
82
55
71
74
69
73
43
57
58
40

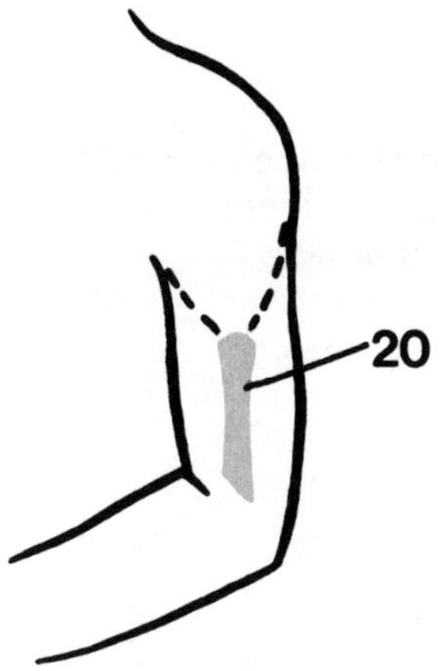
20

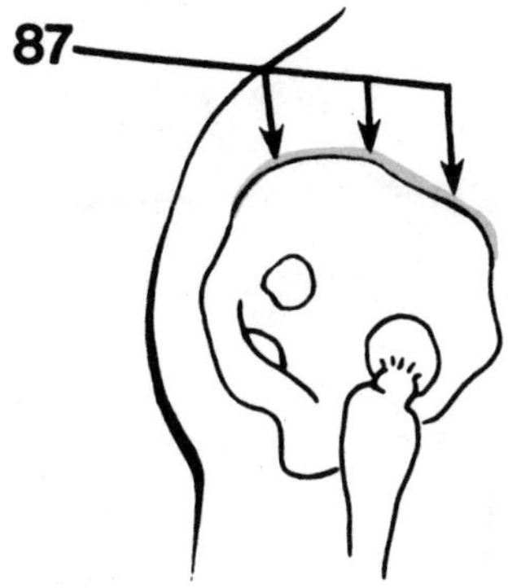
87

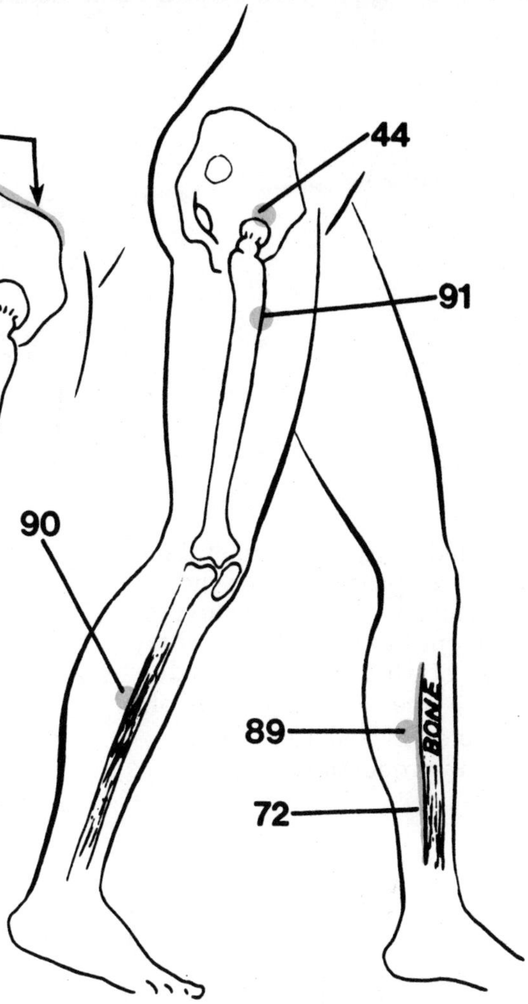
44
91
90
89
BONE
72

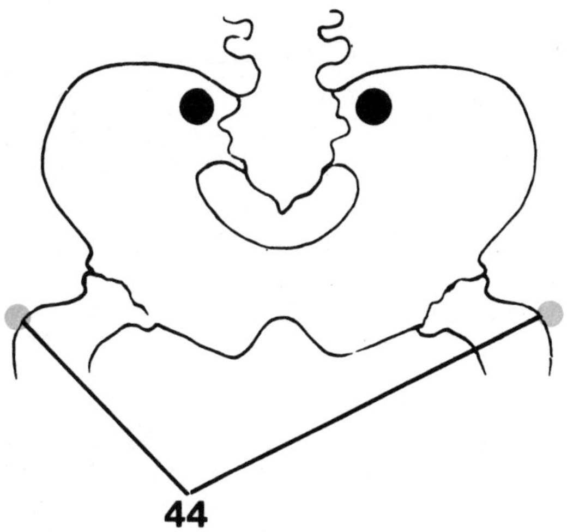
44

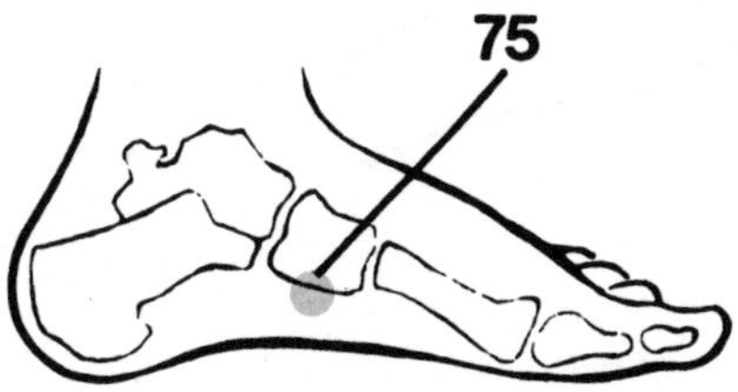
75

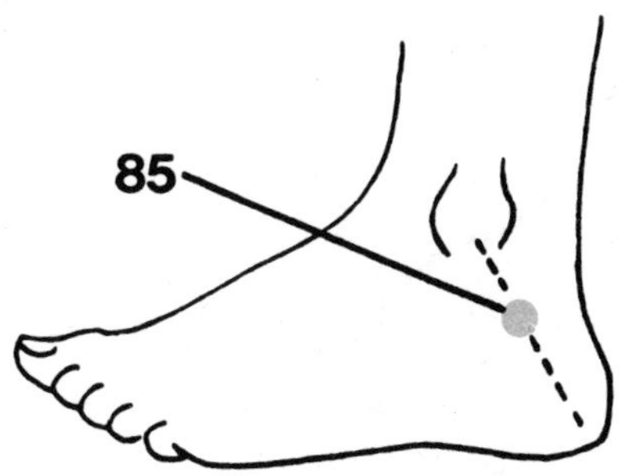
85

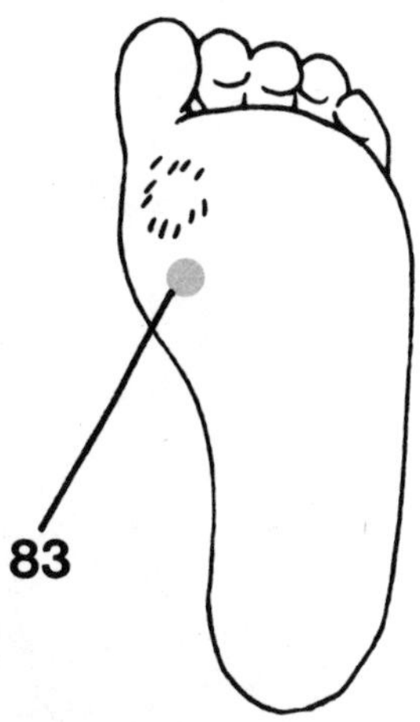
83

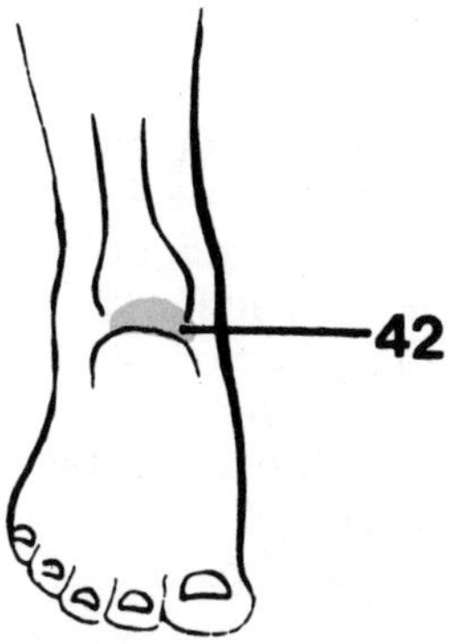
42

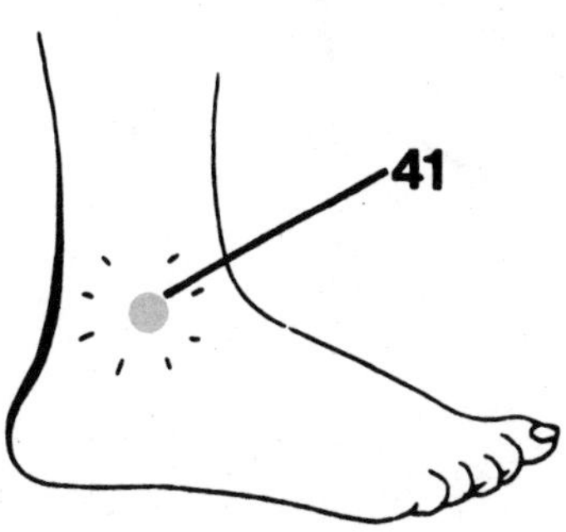
41

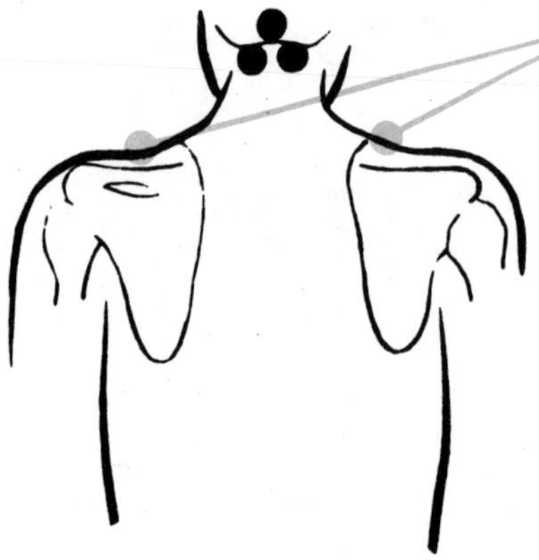

79 energy, tension

Located midway between the base of the neck and shoulders. Treat for tension in shoulders and arms, and also body warmth and energy.

97 sugar control

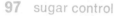

Located beneath the tip of the anconeus process on the end of each elbow. Bend elbow first to find it more easily. These contacts connect with the parathyroid glands and help sugar control, diabetes, hypoglycemia and insulin production.

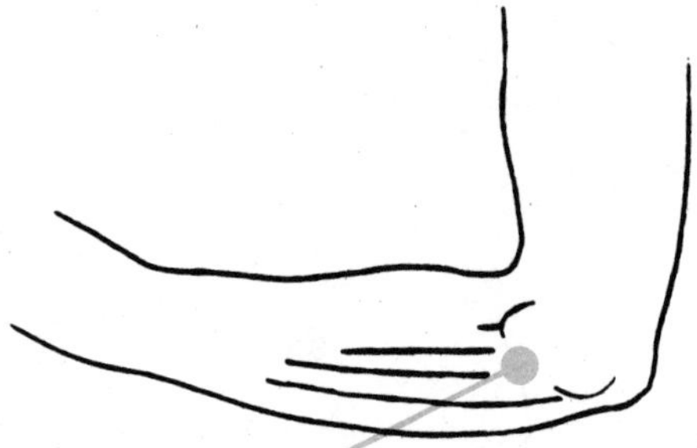

82 circulation of forearms and hands

As shown in the diagram, this contact is at the point on each forearm where the two bones begin to spread apart. These bones are called the radius and ulna and contact on that point controls hand conditions and even goes up into the head. Some anatomy students believe it influences the release of mucous in the body. If #82 contact is painful through to the opposite side of the arm, then treat both sides simultaneously. Helps circulation of forearm and hand.

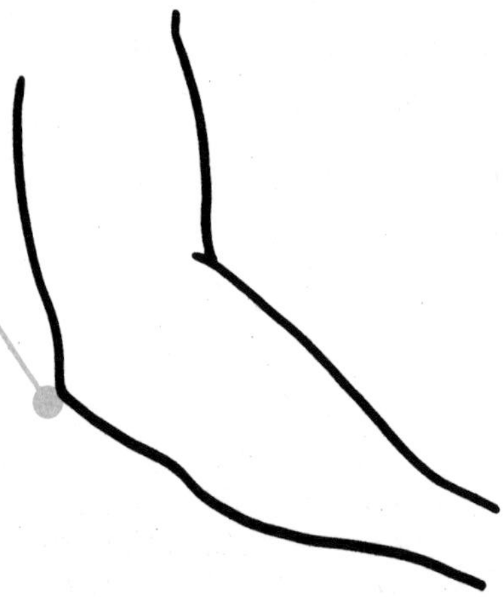

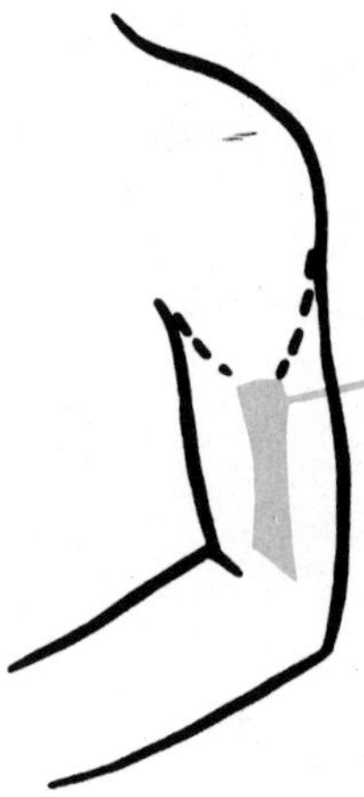

20 arm, neck, head pains, hands, stomach, acid indigestion

Plural contacts on outside aspect of each humerus or upper bone of each arm from elbow to shoulder. Contact must be made on the outside aspect of the bone itself. This treats congestion in the stomach. The left arm contacts the left side of the stomach and the right arm contacts the right side of the stomach. *Note:* stomach trouble can cause severe hand dysfunction. The 20's also help arm, neck and head pains and the hands.

71 colon, leg pains

Located in the center of the heavy calf muscles that form the back of the leg. For pain in the center of this muscle, also for trouble in the colon, or leg pains.

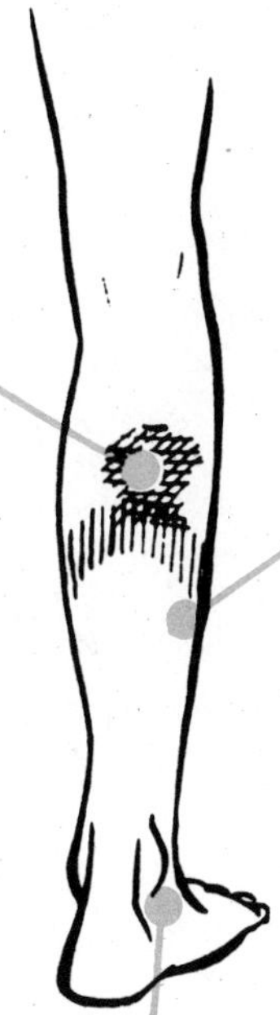

74 muscles

Located on the lateral posterior aspect of the leg muscles. Follow the contour of the muscles downward. Excellent for leg and body muscles.

69 pain, sprains

Located just below each ankle bone on the outside aspect. Contact points are the size of a pea and affect neuralgia, colon, sprains and pain, particularly in the abdomen.

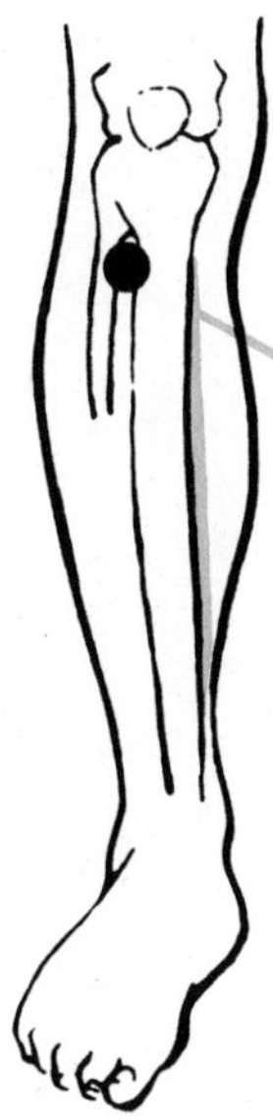

72 colon

Located along the entire medial aspect of the tibia bones of both legs. Contact along these bones treats nerves to the entire colon. Massage only according to tolerance, for even a mild contact can be extremely painful. Very important.

55 intestines

On the inside aspect of each femur or upper leg along its entire length, press in against the bone. This will be painful on nearly everyone since nearly everyone has some sort of eliminative imbalance. These centers treat the intestines.

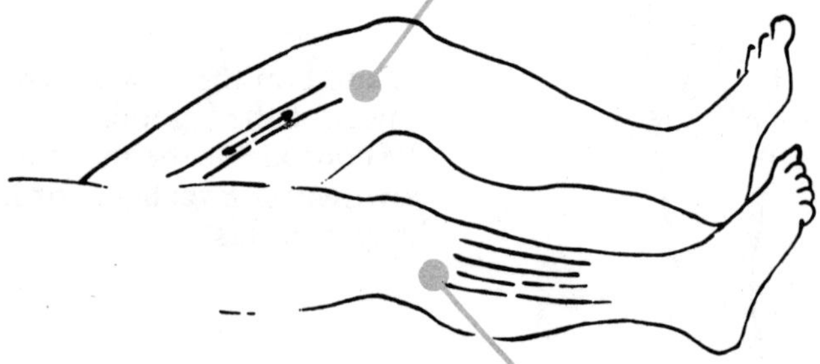

73 abdominal lymph, diabetes, eyes, feet, muscles, thyroid

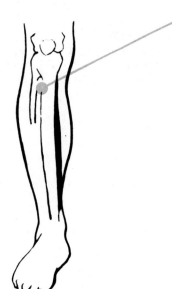

Located at the anterior superior aspect of the legs just at the bifurcation of the tibia and fibula bones. This is the second and most powerful contact to the abdominal lymph. This contact works from the origin of the Achilles tendon back of the heel up the back of the leg to the sacral area where it stimulates the "A" glands in the groin and all the abdominal lymphatic system. Treat for a tonic effect in elderly people; for leg and body muscles; for abdominal bloat; in all cases where the feet are painful and have a burning sensation; for diabetes and thyroid; and for eyes that are painful, degenerating or protruding.

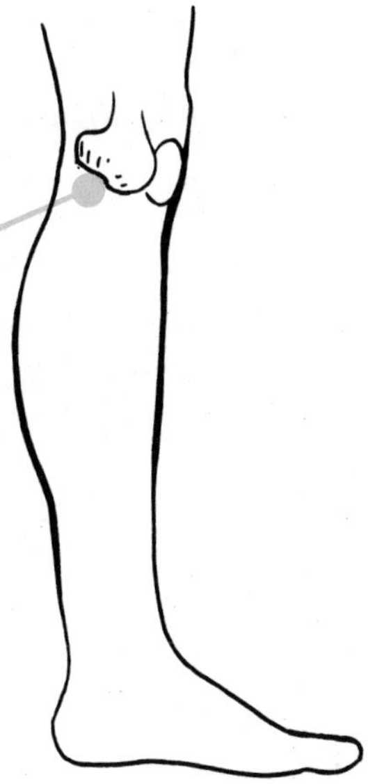

43 abdomen, dizziness, legs

Found on the inner posterior aspect of the condyle, or bone, of each knee. Very important when needed in certain leg (such as the patella or kneecap) and abdominal conditions, particularly having to do with the intestines and spleen. Use also for dizziness.

98 heart lymph, knee dysfunction

The patella or kneecap contacts are located in the soft tissue behind the medial superior crest of each kneecap. Pain on these contacts may indicate malfunction of the patella with subsequent loss of lymph fluid to the heart or dysfunctions of the knee itself.

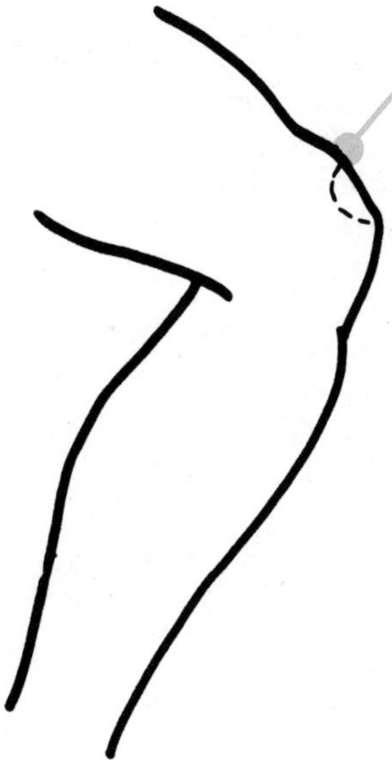

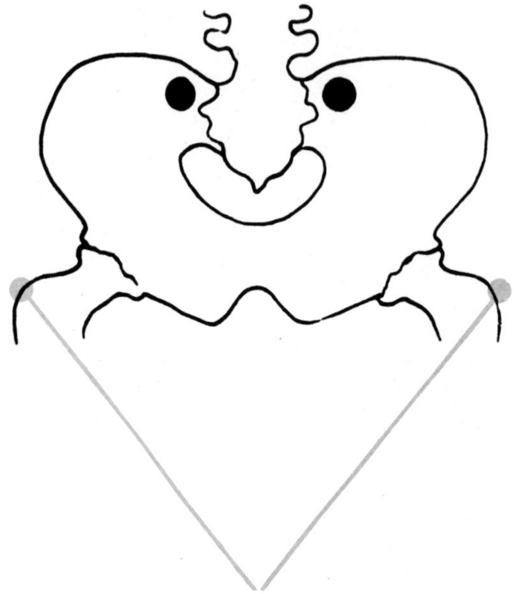

44 constipation, hipbones, intestines, sprains, strains

Formerly a contact on the inside of the thighs against the femur. Now it is the lateral contact on the head or prominence of each greater trochanter. This has long been a contact for strains in any place in the body, but it also treats the hip bones and the intestines. The trochanter is part of the head of the femur, or upper leg bone, and is generally easier for someone else to locate while you are in a seated position. Check these contacts in all constipation cases, and for any sprains or severe strains.

91 colon

In a seated position, press down through the upper leg or thigh until you contact the bone (fairly close to the groin) to help colon.

87 intestines, obesity

This contact is located all along the crest of your hipbones. Check yourself with your thumbs on both hipbones at the same time. Hold those contacts that are painful and you will feel it through your intestines. Since slowness of intestinal function has to do with obesity, use contacts #87 and #44 every day if weight gain is a problem. These contacts also help digestion, and the amino acids.

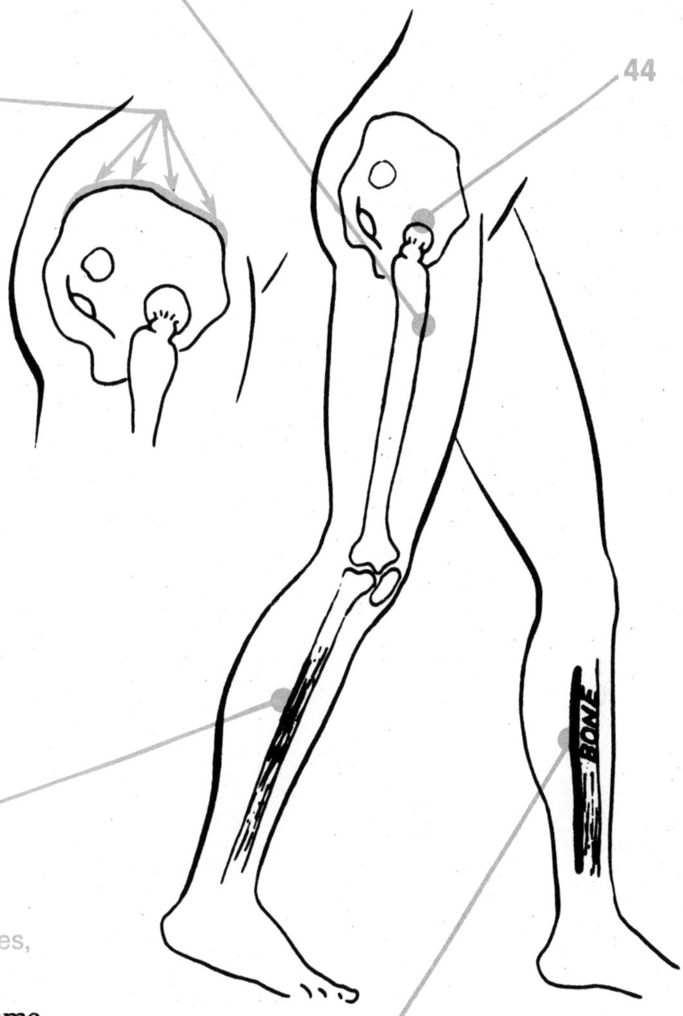

90 hip and leg pains, hormones, tension

Contact is approximately the same as #89 but on the outside aspect of the legs, just behind the tibial bone (shin bone). Press to relax, together with #56 (see page 54) on each side of body, for hip and leg pains and the reproductive hormones.

89 mental confusion, pituitary

Located around the medial aspect of the heavy muscles of the lower legs. If painful, use for the pituitary and "confused thinking." Nearly all young people on drugs will feel pain on this contact.

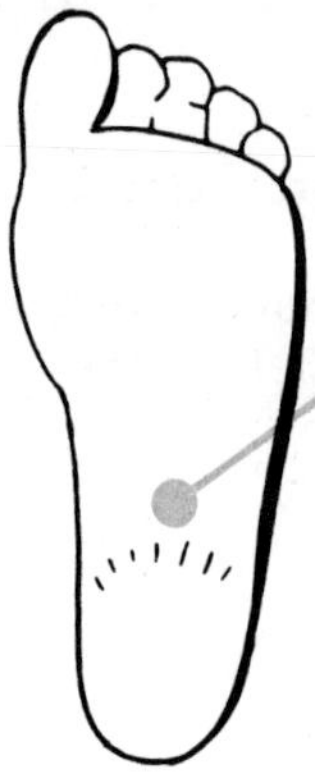

40 energy, inflammation

Located in the center of the bottom of each foot just in front of the heel prominence. These contacts connect energy from the earth to man and can travel clear to the brain. They are very important in all inflammatory conditions, (as #11B for infection) such as colitis, cystitis, peritonitis and phlebitis.

75 breathing, spleen, pancreas

Located against the medial aspect of the foot. Press with the thumb against the metatarsal bones. On both feet the contacts affect the spleen and pancreas and sometimes even breathing.

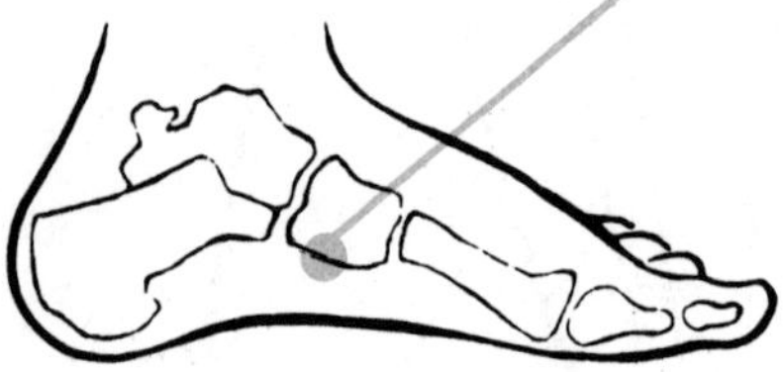

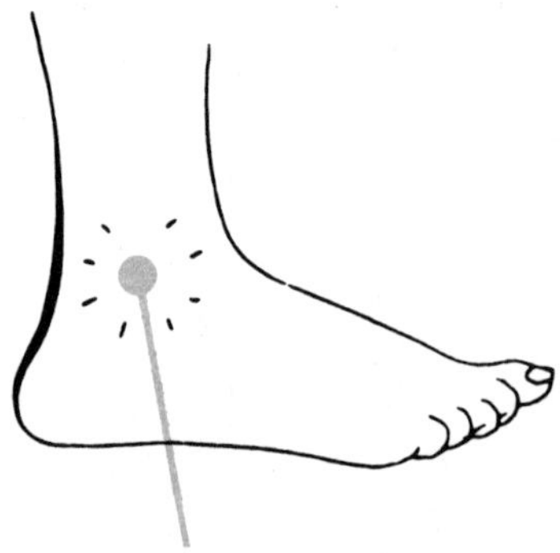

41 ***Systemic***
congestion, constriction, feet, energy

Treat around the ankle bones, both inside and outside of each ankle. Always press from around the outside edge of the ankle bone, in and against it for best results. These contacts seem to be systemic as the reaction can be felt anywhere in the body from head to toes. There is much research yet to be done in this area but remember these contacts for constipation and foot troubles. The inside contacts relate to energy to body tissue; and the outside to congestions and constrictions. Once you begin to treat these centers they become very painful, so use discretion.

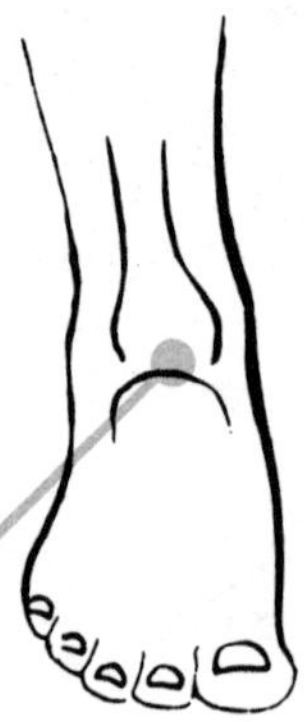

42 eyes

Found in the area between the ankle bone and the tibia or bone of the leg—anterior aspect only. These are direct contacts to eye muscles. Check for pain in this area for all eye troubles.

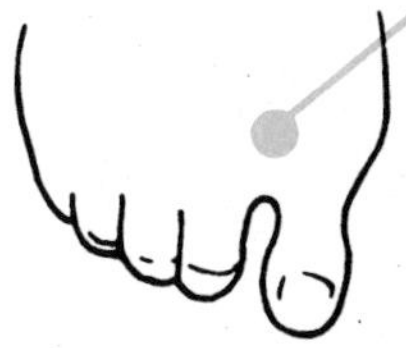

57 bladder and ureter stricture, cramps

With your thumb and index finger, squeeze the tissue between the big toe and the adjacent toe. This is the contact for muscle cramps and cramps or stricture in the opening or outlet of the bladder; also the ureters. (The ureters are the tubes coming down from the kidneys to the bladder.) If there were a kidney stone in the ureter, this contact would be most painful. A stone in this area on the right side would even give the symptoms of appendicitis and the patient would be in great pain. Treat the 57's for tension in both ureters and bladder as well as muscle cramps. (For kidney stones, check #33 [see page 56].)

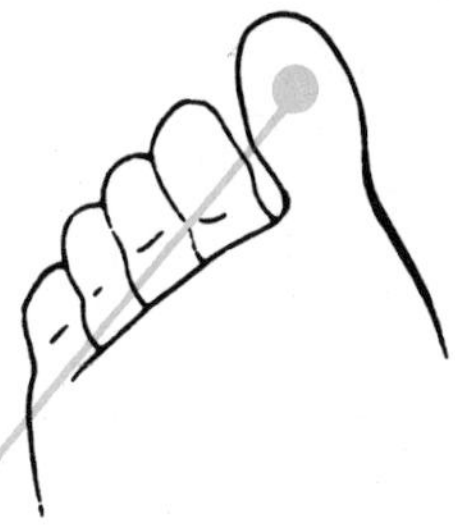

58 breathing, lungs, pituitary

The center of the bottom of the great toes is a reflex contact to the pituitary, as well as to the entire lung structure in certain difficult breathing cases. Treat the 58's and press headward until all slack is taken out of the toes, then hold steady pressure. Breathing is so essential to life we should never forget any contact that will influence it favorably. Flu responds to #58.

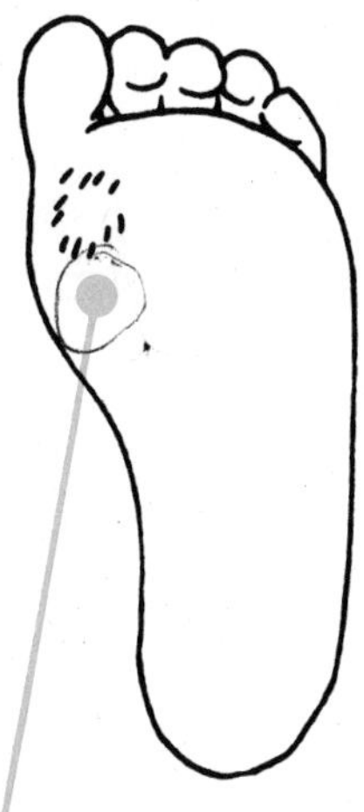

83 bunions, gout, prostate, reproductive organs

This contact is located just posterior to or in back of the prominent joint at the base of the big toe. Slide over the bony prominence, then press in deeply with the end of your thumb to learn if contact is painful. Pain may indicate severe congestion in the reproductive organs; also treat for pain in bunions which may be related.

85 constipation, hipbones, lungs, mucous

At a point midway between the ankle bone and the farthest point on the heel is another contact to the hipbones and lungs. Check for mucous drainage from lungs to the intestines, (#85 contacts should always be checked in constipation as well as lung and hip problems). The contact points are on each side of both feet as shown in diagram. Not as important as #39 (see page 53).

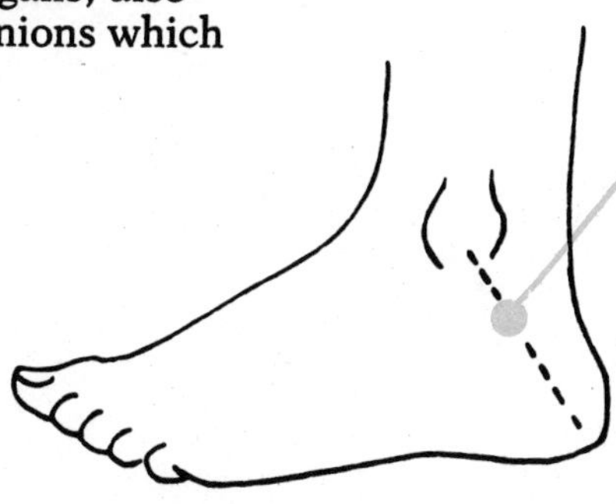

Glossary

Achilles tendon	the strong tendon joining the muscles in the calf of the leg to the bone of the heel
adrenal glands	a pair of complex endocrine organs near the front center border of the kidney that produce sex hormones, metabolic hormones and adrenaline
adrenaline (epinephrine)	a colorless, crystalline hormone used medicinally especially to stimulate the heart, narrow the blood vessels and relax the muscles
anasarca	an abnormal accumulation of serum in the connective tissue
anconeus process	a muscle at the back of the elbow joint, used in extending the forearm
aneurism	a permanent abnormal blood-filled dilatation of a blood vessel resulting from disease of the vessel wall
angina pectoris	a disease condition marked by brief spasms of chest pain precipitated by deficient oxygenation of the heart muscles
anterior	situated before or toward the front
aorta	the great trunk artery that carries blood from the heart to be distibuted by branch arteries through the body
apoplexy	sudden diminution or loss of consciousness, sensation and voluntary motion caused by rupture or obstruction of an artery of the brain
ascites	accumulation of serous fluid in the abdomen
axilla	armpit
bifurcation	branch
bronchi	the two primary divisions of the trachea that lead respectively into the right and the left lung
bursitis	inflammation of a bursa (small serous sac between a tendon and a bone) especially of the shoulder or elbow
capillary	any of the smallest vessels of the blood-vascular system connecting the end-branches of the arteries with minute veins and forming networks throughout the body

carotid	relating to the chief artery or pair of arteries that pass up through the neck and supply the head
cerebellum	a large part of the brain especially concerned with the coordination of muscles and the maintenance of body balance
cerebrum	the expanded front portion of the brain that in higher mammals overlies the rest of the brain, and held to be the seat of conscious mental processes
cervical	relating to the neck or cervix
chyle	lymph that is milky from emulsified fats, characteristically present in the lacteals, vessels which especially carry chyle from the intestines to the thoracic duct
clavicle	the bone which connects the shoulder blade to the breast bone
coccyx	the bottom end of the spine
colitis	inflammation of the colon
colon	extends from the pouch where the large intestine begins to the rectum
condyle	an articular or joint-like prominence on a bone, especially one of a pair, such as knuckles
cranial	relating to the part of the skull that encloses the brain
cystitis	inflammation of the urinary bladder
diplopia	double vision owing to unequal action of the eye muscles
distal	far from the point of attachment or origin
dropsy	an abnormal accumulation of serous fluid in connective tissue or in a serous cavity
duodenum	the first part of the small intestine
dyspepsia	indigestion
eustachian	a bony and cartilaginous tube connecting the middle ear with the upper, or nasal pharynx and equalizing air pressure on both sides of the eardrum
femur	thighbone
fibula	the outer and usually the smaller of the two bones of the leg below the knee
fissure	a natural cleft between body parts or in the substance of an organ; a break in tissue usually at the junction of skin and mucous membrane
fontanelle	a membrane-covered opening at the top of the head where the skull bones do not exactly meet
foramen	a small opening
fossa	an anatomical pit or depression
frontal	relating to the forehead or the frontal bone
glaucoma	a disease of the eye marked by increased pressure within the eyeball, damage to the optic disk and gradual loss of vision
humerus	the long bone of the upper arm extending from the shoulder to the elbow

inferior	situated below a similar superior part
lateral	having to do with the side
lumbar	relating to the part of the back between the ribs and the buttocks
mastoid	a part of the bone behind the ear
maxillary	upper jaw
medulla	the somewhat pyramidal part of the brain where the spinal cord ends
metatarsal	relating to the bones of the foot between the toes and the ankles
occipital	a compound bone at the back of the head that articulates with the first vertebra of the neck
parathyroid	relating to any of four small endocrine glands next to or in the thyroid gland
parietal	the upper rear wall of the head
peritoneum	the smooth transparent serous membrane that lines the cavity of the abdomen
phlebitis	inflammation of a vein
phrenic	relating to the diaphragm
pineal	a small, usually conical appendage of the brain that is said to be a vestigial third eye, an endocrine organ or the seat of the soul
pituitary	relating to a small oval endocrine organ attached to the brain that produces various internal secretions directly or indirectly affecting most basic body functions
pleurisy	inflammation of the pleura (thoracic lining) usually with fever, painful and difficult respiration, cough and exudation into the pleural cavity
plexus	a network of interlacing blood vessels or nerves
pons	a broad mass of nerve fibers lying across the front surface of the brain
portal	a large vein that collects blood from one part of the body and distributes it in another part through a capillary network
posterior	or dorsal; near or on the back
prominence	a part that juts out
ptosis	a sagging of an organ or part
pylorus	the opening from the stomach to the intestine
sacrum	the part of the vertebral column that forms a part of the pelvis and consists of five united vertebrae
sciatic	situated near the hip, or relating to sciatica, a pain along the sciatic nerve
sigmoid	the contracted and crooked part of the colon immediately above the rectum
solar plexus	a network of interlacing nerves in the abdomen behind the stomach and in front of the aorta
spinous	bony part of the arch enclosing the spinal cord on the back side of the vertebra

sternocleidomastoid	belonging to the sternum, the clavicle and the mastoid process
styloid	the slender, pointed projecting part of bones, as on the temporal bone or ulna
superior	situated above, in front of or in back of another and especially corresponding part
supraclavicular	situated above the clavicle
supraorbital	situated above the bony socket of the eye
sylvian fissure	a deep, narrow depression dividing the front and middle lobes of the cerebrum on each side
systemic	affecting the body generally
temporal bone	compound bone of the side of the skull
thalamus	a large, ovoid mass of grey matter situated at the base of the brain and involved in the transmission and integration of certain sensations
thoracic duct	the main trunk of the system of lymphatic vessels lying along the front of the spinal column
thorax	the part of the body between the neck and the abdomen
thymus	a glandular structure of uncertain function that is present in the young of most vertebrates in the upper chest or at the base of the neck which tends to disappear or become rudimentary in the adult
thyroid	a large endocrine lying at the base of the neck and producing an iodine-containing hormone that especially affects growth, development and metabolic rate
tibia	the inner and usually larger of the two bones of the back of the leg between the knee and the ankle
tinnitus	a sensation of noise in the ear
trachea	the main trunk of the system of tubes by which air passes to and from the lungs
trochanter	a rough prominence at the upper part of the thighbone
vagus	either of the tenth pair of cranial nerves arising from the medulla and supplying the viscera with autonomic sensory and motor fibers
varicosities	the state of being abnormally swollen or dilated

Index

Legend:

JB — Jawbone
S — Breast contacts
E — Ear treatment
X's — Blood
MB — Double contact

Systemic Contacts:

25	78	21	LT-X
19's	63	13B	5M's
10M's	1B	2B	15M's
62	49	64	RT-X

Where to Find Pressure Points